The Juice Lady's

ANTI-INFLAMMATION
DIET

The Juice Lady's

ANTI-INFLAMMATION
DIET

Cherie Calbom, MS, CN

With Chef Abby Fammartino

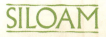

Most CHARISMA HOUSE BOOK GROUP products are available at special quantity discounts for bulk purchase for sales promotions, premiums, fund-raising, and educational needs. For details, write Charisma House Book Group, 600 Rinehart Road, Lake Mary, Florida 32746, or telephone (407) 333-0600.

THE JUICE LADY'S ANTI-INFLAMMATION DIET by Cherie Calbom
    with Abby Fammartino
Published by Siloam
Charisma Media/Charisma House Book Group
600 Rinehart Road
Lake Mary, Florida 32746
www.charismahouse.com

Cover design by Justin Evans

Visit the author's website at www.juiceladycherie.com.

Library of Congress Control Number: 2014957629
International Standard Book Number: 978-1-62998-002-7
E-book ISBN: 978-1-62998-003-4

This book contains the opinions and ideas of its author. It is solely for informational and educational purposes and should not be regarded as a substitute for professional medical treatment. The nature of your body's health condition is complex and unique. Therefore, you should consult a health professional before you begin any new exercise, nutrition, or supplementation program or if you have questions about your health. Neither the author nor the publisher shall be liable or responsible for any loss or damage allegedly arising from any information or suggestion in this book.

Meal recipes and some snack and dessert recipes contributed by Chef Abby.

16 17 18 19 20 — 9 8 7 6 5 4
Printed in the United States of America

CONTENTS

2 FOODS AND FACTORS THAT CONTRIBUTE TO INFLAMMATION 15

3   CHANGE YOUR DIET; CHANGE YOUR LIFE!....29

4 TWENTY-EIGHT DAYS TO VIBRANT HEALTH RECIPES AND MEAL PLAN................................57

CHERIE CALBOM'S INFORMATION 213

CHEF ABBY FAMMARTINO AND ABBY'S TABLE INFORMATION.. 217

RECIPES

Juices

Smoothies

Teas

Breakfast/Brunch

Lunch

Chicken

Seafood

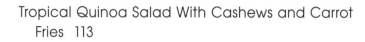

Dinner

Chicken

Seafood

Vegetarian/Vegan

Salads

Soups

Side Dishes

Dressings, Marinades, Sauces, and Seasoning

Snacks

Desserts

Introduction

YOUR DIET PLAN FOR VIBRANT HEALTH

The first wealth is health.[1]
—RALPH WALDO EMERSON

THERE ARE MANY factors in our modern lifestyle that pull us away from the health we want, the health we need to complete our purpose. In this book you'll read about a number of factors that contribute to disease and inflammation. Of all of them, diet is undoubtedly number one for most people in Western countries. Because our food has changed so drastically in recent decades, many people no longer eat fresh, local, organic, and seasonal foods served up with love and care in preparation. We're flying down life's fast lane grabbing convenience food as we go. The result is a laundry list of ailments that plague our nation. This fast, convenient food is causing inflammation, which is at the root of disease. It's destroying the health and lives of many people. Because inflammation is a major challenge, I've devoted this book to the discussion of this chronic problem and the lifestyle to overcome it. *The Juice Lady's Anti-Inflammation Diet* gives you four weeks of great-tasting recipes that are not only anti-inflammatory but are also designed to nourish and bring enjoyment for you and your family and friends.

A Personal Note From Cherie

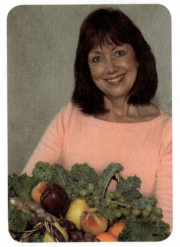

Many people ask me what they should eat in addition to their juices and green smoothies. I often say *an anti-inflammatory diet*. They nearly always ask where they can find that. And for people who have inflammation and must eat this type of diet to recover, a good meal plan with recipes is imperative. Hence, the inspiration for this book was born.

Maybe you or a loved one has dealt with pain, eczema, obesity, attention deficit disorder (ADD), attention deficit hyperactivity disorder (ADHD), peripheral neuropathy, diabetes, heart disease, stroke, migraines, thyroid problems, dental issues, cancer, or another illness or disease. If you have, you've dealt with inflammation. One of the important ways to heal the body, whatever you may suffer, is to eat a diet that does not promote inflammation, along with making lifestyle changes such as stress reduction, maintaining a positive attitude, and practicing love and appreciation.

Where do you start in making healing dietary changes? Choose whole food minus the pro-inflammatory fare, grown locally without pesticides, and prepared at home. It might take a little practice to learn how to make good food, but it's worth every effort. And once you get the hang of it, preparing delicious food should bring you lots of pleasure.

I first fell in love with preparing whole food when I was a child. One of my father's great joys in life was to cook. He got excited about the food he made. He often brought all the kids of our extended family together in the kitchen on holidays to taste his turkey and dressing before it went to the table. I thoroughly enjoyed preparing food beside him, and I never lost my joy of cooking. That is perhaps why I ended up cooking with the George Foreman Grill for thirteen years on QVC and demonstrating the Juiceman juicer all across America.

My grandmother instilled in me a love for the earth and growing things. She had a bountiful garden that she tended with love and pride well into her eighties. Then it was just called *eating home-grown food*. Today the popular term is farm to table. That was nothing chic or exotic in my parents or grandparent's day; it was simply how people ate ... real whole food grown without chemicals or genetically modified foods, picked fresh or canned for winter, and prepared in the kitchen. It was the only way most people ate for centuries. The desire to grow food is deep within my soul, and it's why I always grow pots of tomatoes and herbs every year.

But I lost my way in my teens, and that carried over into my twenties when it came to food choices. I started eating boatloads of fast food and sweets; I didn't like vegetables. My health took a dive, and I ended up with chronic fatigue syndrome and fibromyalgia. Doctors gave me no hope of recovery. I knew I had to find my own way. My healing journey began with a five-day vegetable juice fast and a summer of strictly juices, vegetables, and brown rice. I was completely well in three months. I recovered because I gave my body what it needed to heal and detoxify. That's why I'm passionate about helping you find the path to good health too.

We started losing our way as a nation in the 1950s. The lure of time-saving modern appliances and the fascination with the television made way for Gerry Thomas's TV dinners. More than 10 million Swanson TV dinners were sold during the first year of national distribution. Had it not been for Julia Child who revolutionized the way women viewed cooking, many of us may never have eaten anything again but a TV dinner and food from a box. Nevertheless, the concept of fast food was here to stay. Slick marketing made women believe they had no time to prepare a meal from scratch, and they had to find food that was either fast to make or take home. That era ushered in the slippery slope of refined foods and ill health. Food became focused on task rather than nutrition.

After many hours in my nutrition practice of counseling people with a variety of illnesses and diseases—all with inflammation at the root—I knew I needed a healing diet plan and interesting recipes for people to follow. But I also realized that many people are not comfortable in the kitchen and need help learning some basics of making good food. I thought about Abby, who for years sent me beautiful menu plans and recipes via her "Abby's Table" e-newsletter. I first met Chef Abby when she made a beautiful food presentation at one of my raw foods parties in my home. Her recipe creations are delicious. Pictures of her food are beautiful.

I invited her to coauthor this book. We teamed up to bring you a wide variety of healthy, scrumptious recipes and menu plans designed with your health and healing in mind. I've written the opening chapters to give you information on inflammation, the factors that contribute to it, and the foods that help you get it under control or prevent it from flaring up in the first place. I'm pleased to present our twenty-eight-day plan that includes juices, green smoothies, and a wide variety of health-enhancing recipes complete with lovely pictures and shopping lists.

I hope you're inspired by each meal and enjoy the benefits of eating healthy food—food that loves you back.

Cherie Calbom
THE JUICE LADY
health, healing and wholeness

A Personal Note From Chef Abby

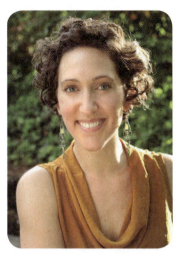

My recipes are a jumping off point for learning useful, healthful cooking techniques for all types of eaters. Over the last ten years and counting, I've devoted my life to making inspiring food the body loves. I've run a supper club, created a commercial sauce line, cooked on a boat for forty days, cooked for individuals in their home, taught classes of all kinds for kids and adults, and cooked for hundreds of celebrations of life, love, and hard work. I've also dedicated various dinners, lectures, and classes to sharing foods that suit the seasons, teaching people the wonders (and everyday ease) of treating food as medicine. In culinary school we learned a great deal about the Chinese Five Phase theory as it relates to seasonal eating for optimal health. Through it all my mission is to build community around vibrant, health-giving food. Bringing everyone's health needs to the table, I work to make healthy food fun, social, and practical for everyday life.

All my recipes are naturally gluten, dairy, and soy free and are suitable for an anti-inflammatory diet. By reducing overall consumption of common food allergens and inflaming foods, you do your body a favor. Food sensitivities, much like seasonal allergies, can be kept at bay if your overall consumption level is low and you do not experience life-threatening reactions.

Imagine a glass of water; as you fill the glass with more water, at some point the glass begins to overflow and spill out onto the table. Similarly, when your body is overloaded with foods that cause inflammation (such as refined sugar, wheat, or dairy), you start to feel symptomatic. Sluggishness, fogginess, bloating, and depression can be greatly reduced by enjoying a diet consisting largely of naturally allergen-free whole foods. Fortunately for us, a whole-foods-based diet rich in seasonal produce, high quality meat, and wild fish can provide infinite inspiration and satisfying flavor.

In my work I love to bring people together around a table to celebrate great food. For my supper club events, eaters of all kinds enjoy a family style meal together where no one is the odd man out for eating the foods that support their health. I host these events in interesting venues in Portland and now across the country. I also teach private cooking lessons for groups of friends, family, or coworkers in the comfort of their homes. This is where true kitchen confidence is born—in the home kitchen. In these lessons my goal is to connect the cooks with how food supports overall life and how important (and fun!) it is to bring loved ones to the table for this purpose.

To truly reap the benefits of a naturally healthy diet, it's crucial to get in the kitchen and just start cooking. Find ways to cook every day. The more you practice, the more fun and relaxing it will be.

—ABBY

Chapter 1

INFLAMMATION: FRIEND OR FOE

Chronic inflammation is the evil mother of the most preva-
lent and devastating diseases that routinely kill Americans.[1]
—Dr. Barry Sears

SUDDENLY INFLAMMATION HAS become one of the hottest interests of medical research. Barely a week goes by without another study revealing a new way chronic inflammation does harm to the body. Cholesterol deposits are destabilized in the coronary arteries, leading to heart attacks and potentially strokes. It devours nerve cells in the brains of Alzheimer's victims. It can foster the proliferation of abnormal cells and facilitate their transformation into cancer. Chronic inflammation may be the engine that drives the majority of the most feared illnesses of middle and old age.

Though you may not have a warm, fuzzy feeling about it, inflammation is a natural response to trauma, infection, disease, and other physical assaults. It helps to rid the body of bacteria and toxins. It also "mops up" dead cells and tissues. Without inflammation, injured tissues would not heal and infections would flame out of control.

Chronic inflammation, however, is not a good response. It's an inflammatory immune response of prolonged duration that eventually leads to tissue damage. It's low grade and systemic. It can have a domino effect that can seriously damage your health. The root cause of many illnesses is chronic inflammation—a lingering immune response caused by poor diet, allergic reactions, stress, toxins, and/or psychological issues. If it is left unchecked, it can damage many important systems, including the endocrine (hormone), immune, digestive, cardiovascular, and respiratory systems.

One of the most destructive inflammatory molecules, called nuclear factor kappa B, is a little molecule that creates significant damage in the body. Emotional stress, toxins, free radicals, and toxic, inflammatory, or allergenic foods can activate it. When it is set off, it can unleash the production of numerous inflammatory molecules—a steamroller of inflammation that affects the entire body. It might show up in a finger joint, your knees, your arteries, or your heart.

It is estimated that more than half of all Americans are inflamed, with most of them not even knowing they are. Most ailments are associated with chronic inflammation, such as heart disease, lupus, rheumatoid arthritis, fibromyalgia, atherosclerosis, inflammatory bowel disease, chronic pancreatitis, and chronic hepatitis. New research also links obesity with inflammation. Being overweight promotes inflammation and inflammation promotes obesity—a continuous and frustrating cycle.

These conditions and many more arise from an immune system that is out of control. It affects you at the cellular level. Even the mitochondria can be inflamed. When symptoms of inflammation don't abate, the message is that your immune system is stuck in the "on" position—even when you aren't in imminent danger. When the rhythm of the immune system is disrupted, it shifts into a continual state of alarm, with inflammation spreading rapidly throughout the body. When the inflammation "alarm" sounds in the heart, it causes heart disease; in the brain, dementia or Alzheimer's disease; in the eyes, disorders such as macular degeneration; and in the fat cells, obesity. It is also a major contributor to obesity.

Our bodies weren't designed for a daily barrage of toxins, infectious agents, genetically modified food, pesticide-sprayed food, refined foods, or intense, prolonged stress. This kind of demand requires significant support to maintain the immune system's resilience. Our on-the-go lifestyle doesn't lean toward immune support unless we pay particular attention to everything we do—what we breathe, eat, drink, think, and feel.

While the incidence of inflammation and inflammatory disease is rising in all developed countries, we are not stuck with this scenario. We have a choice in how we respond to the stressors in our life, along with what we choose to eat and drink, and how we think. Some of our responses are learned behavior from our earliest days. However, changing our responses to life's stressors and what we eat and drink is within our control. We can make positive responses and choices.

CHOLESTEROL, INFLAMMATION, AND HEART DISEASE

Have you ever wondered if plaque buildup in the circulatory system is the real culprit in heart disease since people are popping cholesterol-lowering drugs like candy and heart disease is still the number one killer? Rather than the villain, cholesterol is the healing agent the body sends to sites to cover the lesions in blood vessels that have been caused by inflammation. If you have too much cholesterol buildup in your arteries, the problem is too much inflammation rather than too much cholesterol. Your body is not in need of a drug; you need to get inflammation under control.

"It's the inflammation in the vessels that starts the lesion," says Dr. Beverly Teter, a lipid biochemist from the University of Maryland who has been researching fats and their effect on the human body for many years. "The body then sends the cholesterol like a scab to cover over it to protect the blood system and the vessel wall from further damage."[2]

Americans have been duped into taking cholesterol-lowering drugs and avoiding high-quality fats like coconut oil to their own demise, while they gorge on oxidized vegetable oils, trans fats, sugar, grains, and low-fat junk foods—the real contributors to inflammation and heart disease.

Is Your System Stuck on "Slow Simmer" or a "Bubbling Boil"?

With inflammation turning up the heat inside your body, you may develop a host of symptoms such as high triglycerides, high cholesterol, dry skin, swollen tissues and joints, weight gain, and an agitated response to life's challenges and stresses.

Many people in this country experience prolonged "slow simmer" inflammation—a major setup for health problems. We have billowing rates of heart disease, cancer, allergies, asthma, diabetes, obesity, irritable bowel syndrome (IBS), and chronic pain just to name a few of the conditions caused by inflammation. There's such a spike in inflammatory symptoms that it's becoming the norm rather than the exception. Some people have such raging inflammation they're in "rolling boil." But there is good news. Once we understand what causes it and see how quickly our actions can either fan the flame or cool the internal fire, we can make better choices each day that bring us back into balance.

IT'S NOT WISE TO RELY ON NONSTEROIDAL ANTI-INFLAMMATORY DRUGS

Here's what's associated with NSAIDS:

- 3,300 deaths per year
- 41,000 hospitalizations a year
- Gastrointestinal (GI) bleeding
- Cardiovascular risk
- Leads to gut dysbiosis, which worsens inflammation[3]

An Unhappy Gut

Babies who are not born by C-section and have been breast fed have healthier gut bacteria. Many people were not breast fed and consequently have more health challenges. Also, taking antibiotics kills good bacteria and sets you up for overgrowth of yeast and other pathogens. Sugars feed the yeast, causing it to get out of control.

Problems usually start in the gut—bloating, frequent bouts of diarrhea or constipation, gas, belching, heartburn, and acid reflux—all indicating an inflamed intestinal tract. The immune system goes into action when we eat inflammatory foods because it was designed to seek and destroy threatening substances such as viruses, parasites, and bacteria in our food. Our digestive system has to extract the nutrients from the inflammatory and useless matter that we eat and then get rid of or store the rest.

Most people in the Western Hemisphere overwork their digestive system because a large portion of what they eat is inflammatory to the intestinal tract. Our ancestors hunted and gathered their food—real, whole food the body could use. Today we consume large quantities of convenience, refined, and fast foods, which overwhelm the body and create a damaged gut.

AILMENTS AND DISEASES INVOLVING INFLAMMATION*

Acne	Acrodermatitis
Actinic keratosis	Alzheimer's disease
Amyloidosis	Ankylosing spondylitis
Arthritis	Atherosclerosis (hardening of the arteries)
Bursitis	Cancer
Candidiasis	Celiac
Cellulitis	Cerebrovascular disease
Cervicitis	Chronic fatigue syndrome
Colitis	Common cold
Crohn's disease	Cystitis
Decubitus ulcer	Dermatomyositis
Diabetes mellitus	Eczema

* This is not an exhaustive list but is meant to give you an idea of all the diseases where inflammation is involved.

AILMENTS AND DISEASES INVOLVING INFLAMMATION

Fungal nail infection	Gastritis
GERD	Gout
Grave's disease	Heart disease
Hemangioma of skin	Hepatitis
Herpetic stomatitis	HIV/AIDS
Hives	Hypohidrosis
Ichthyosis vulgaris	Impetigo
Inflammatory bowel disease	Inflammatory conditions of the skin
Inflammatory diseases of the joints	Inflammatory heart disease
Inflammatory vascular diseases	Impetigo
Ischemic heart disease	Juvenile arthritis
Kaposi sarcoma	Lichen planus
Lumbar spinal stenosis	Lupus
Metabolic syndrome	Multiple sclerosis
Necrotizing fasciitis	Nephritis
Neurodegenerative diseases	Neurotropic viral infections
Osteoarthritis	Osteoporosis
Paraneoplastic syndromes	Parkinson's disease
Pelvic inflammatory diseases	Pilonidal cyst
Prostatitis	Psoriasis
Psoriatic arthritis	Reactive arthritis
Rheumatoid arthritis	Rheumatic heart disease
Rosacea	Sacroiliac joint pain
SAPHO syndrome	Sarcoidosis
Schleraderma	Seborrheic eczema
Seborrheic keratosis	Sexually transmitted infections
Sinuitis	Shingles
Sickle cell disease	Skin cancer
Stasis dermatitis	Still's Disease

AILMENTS AND DISEASES INVOLVING INFLAMMATION	
Stroke	Systemic inflammatory diseases
Systemic vasculitis	Tendonitis
Tinea versicolor	Ulcerative colitis
Vaginitis	Vitiligo

An Inflammatory Lifestyle

Otherwise healthy individuals can be exposed through lifestyle and/or environment to substances the body perceives as irritants, such as infections, viruses, parasites or bacteria, food allergens, toxins, and inflammatory foods such as sugar, artificial sweeteners, alcohol, oxidized oils, gluten, dairy, and MSG. The causes of chronic inflammation can vary person to person, but include being overweight, experiencing stress, eating bad food, and breathing polluted air. Lifestyle choices such as smoking or lack of exercise also play a role. A sedentary lifestyle and lack of sleep can also increase long-term inflammation. However, one of the biggest factors is the inflammatory foods we eat.

Factors Contributing to Chronic Inflammation

Psychological factors

Have you ever watched a scary movie with your heart pounding? Reactions like this initiated by a perceived threat (real or fictional) dilate your blood vessels—just like inflammation. Wider capillaries mean more blood and nutrients get to your organs to help you fight off an attack or deal with a threat. This is the "fight or flight" response. It triggers the release of the stress hormone cortisol from your adrenal glands with a cascade of other stress hormones, including adrenaline and norepinephrine.

A duck may be cruising on a lake and encounter a threatening situation. It quacks, walks out of the lake, flaps its wings, and flies away. The stress is over. You may have a near accident driving home from work, and the stress effects could last a couple of days before you can let it go and move on. When you stew about a problem, the body continuously releases cortisol day after day, week after week. Too much cortisol can suppress the immune system, increase blood pressure, elevate blood sugar, decrease libido, produce acne, deposit fat on the midsection, keep you awake at night, and contribute to obesity. Cortisol has a direct role in chronic inflammation.

How many times have you seen this response in your life? You work endless hours preparing for a test, a presentation, or your vacation and then get sick. Your body is good at keeping things under control for a while, but it can't do that forever. Dealing with persistent stress takes a toll on your immune system, your adrenal and thyroid glands, your central nervous system...and your entire body.

Research has linked depression and stress to a rise in inflammatory markers such as C-reactive protein (CRP). This is a test that measures the concentration in blood serum of a special type of protein produced in the liver, which is elevated during episodes of acute inflammation or infection. An elevated CRP test result is an indicator of acute inflammation. This is a primary indicator of a potential risk for heart disease (not high cholesterol). About as many people die of heart attacks with low cholesterol as with high cholesterol.

Your body reacts to stressors in a general manner regardless of what they are. The more serious the threat appears, the more dramatic the response will be. With inflammation, painful emotional experiences are as harmful as physical stress or inflammatory foods. Consider a condition like asthma. An emotional shock can trigger an asthma attack in some people as quickly as physical exertion or an allergen. Thoughts and feelings are powerful. They manifest themselves physically with inflammatory symptoms. Emotional stress can cause your skin to break out and your intestinal track to go haywire. But here's the good news: your emotions and your mind can be your allies in the healing process as well. It all depends on how you choose to react in various situations.

You can let go of toxic emotions such as anger, resentment, rejection from others, self-rejection, worry, fear, and bitterness. You can enter into a place of peace with yourself and others. This is as important as eating an anti-inflammatory diet if you want to get rid of chronic inflammation.

Your daily expressions may hold some clues to your inner world of emotions. How often do you use words such as *hopping mad*, *burned out*, *fed up*, *sick and tired*, *worried sick*, or *afraid it won't work out?* The conflicts within your body and soul release powerful inflammatory hormones, acid in your stomach, and pain in your head, joints, and muscles. They are there to tell you there's a problem. The solution is letting go of negative emotions and thoughts, making peace with yourself and others, and choosing joy, peace, love, trust, and acceptance. Also, a physical exercise program that produces feel-good endorphins will help your body control inflammation.

Managing emotional pain is often overlooked, but it is an important component you can address in alleviating inflammation. This can also play a big part in restoring your immune system's balance.

> Research shows that oxytocin reduces levels of free radicals and inflammation and so slows aging and disease at the root level. Oxytocin is a neurohypophysial hormone that is secreted by the posterior pituitary gland. It acts primarily as a neuromodulator in the brain. Acts of kindness are often accompanied by emotional warmth, and emotional warmth produces oxytocin in the brain and throughout the body. Also, references in scientific journals indicate a strong link between compassion and the activity of the vagus nerve. The vagus nerve controls inflammation levels in the body.[4]

Stress

When you have endless housecleaning and company coming or project deadlines that appear impossible to meet, you have a choice. You can allow yourself to get worked into a frenzy, or you can choose to relax even in the midst of the fray. You can let go. Believe me, I know this firsthand. I used to get so worked up over book deadlines, I couldn't even sleep at night. I've written twenty-six books, so I've had a few sleepless nights. This significantly slowed down my work. Stressful responses don't have positive outcomes. You can choose to work as efficiently as possible and trust that it will all come together. As you learn to relax and let go of stress, you can live harmoniously regardless of the stressors. This will help you work and interact with people more creatively and efficiently. That is a big factor in managing stress. "Want to" rather than "should" or "have to" is a big stress reducer as well. *Shoulds* don't work anyway; they just contribute to stress. When you want to do something, when you feel you have a choice in the matter and how you design your time, you have more control and less stress.

Stress is a huge contributing factor to inflammation. It is responsible for harmful chemicals that flood your body. Stress hormones are acidic, which can damage your cells. Stress also affects your brain neurotransmitters, causing your excitatory transmitters such as norepinephrine to rise and calming transmitters such as serotonin to drop. Then your mind starts chattering in the evening when you need to sleep and can keep you awake half the night. An exhaustive discussion of stress is far beyond the scope of this book but extremely important to explore. If you were to talk with my psychotherapist husband, he would tell you it's a major contributor to inflammation and disease. This short section won't solve your stress issues, but I hope to inspire you to seek help with your stress and get it managed.

Stress will always be a part of life. We can't avoid it. But whether it destroys our lives or not depends wholly on our responses to it.

Poor sleep

Those who have insomnia secrete inflammatory cytokines at a higher rate compared to those who do not. During sleep the body regenerates, healing hormones are released, and the immune system calms down and is able to rejuvenate. Lack of restorative sleep is a major promoter of inflammation. People who suffer with pain know this firsthand, because lack of sleep due to pain is associated with flare-ups and more pain. There is help for insomnia. Here are some factors to explore:

- Adrenal imbalance. To determine your adrenal stress level, you can take my Adrenal Health Quiz at http://www.juiceladycherie.com/Juice/do-you-have-adrenal-fatigue/. If you have a high score, I recommend my book *The Juice Lady's Remedies for Stress and Adrenal Fatigue*. If your adrenals are low, this could keep you awake at night. You can also order the saliva test to determine just how stressed your adrenal glands are at www.neurogistics.com. Use my practitioner code SLEEP (all caps).

- Anxiety, worry, or troubled thoughts. You must find a way to get all this out of your mind and soul at night, or you won't sleep well. Again, this is beyond the scope of this book but extremely important to address.

- Brain neurotransmitter imbalance. The amino acid program I work with to balance brain chemistry has been very helpful for many people, along with stress reduction. You can order a urinalysis test that will give you a print out of the status of your neurotransmitters and a recommendation of the amino acids that will help you bring them into balance. You can order the urinalysis test at www.neurogistics.com. Use my practitioner code SLEEP (all caps).

- Nutrient imbalances. You may be magnesium deficient. If this mineral is low, it can cause you to wake up during the night. If calcium is low, it can keep you from falling asleep. Also, consuming sweets, caffeine, or drinking too much alcohol can disturb your sleep.

Environmental toxicity

Synthetics, latex, glues, dyes, adhesives, plastics, air fresheners, and toxic cleaning products all represent chemicals we are exposed to frequently. Many of us work in office buildings, plants, or airplanes with recirculated air that only increases our exposure to environmental toxins.

Have you heard of "sick building syndrome"? The term is used to describe building occupants who experience acute health and comfort issues that are linked to time spent in toxic buildings, and just as sick buildings make people sick, so do pesticides, pollution, and heavy metals such as lead, cadmium, and mercury. These heavy metals are just three of more than two dozen heavy metals in our environment that our bodies must try to detoxify. Toxins are everywhere: our drinking water, our food, our air, and even mothers' breast milk. Many of these chemicals are fat soluble, which means they are stored in fat cells and tissue spaces until they reach damaging levels.

Chemical sensitivity is not the only result of this noxious mix of harmful substances. Constant exposure to toxic chemicals and airborne irritants, even in low doses, makes your immune system go haywire. Some people are better detoxifiers than others and can withstand more exposure before they show symptoms. Others need health support early on in their lives. Learn as much as you can about the beauty, cleaning, and gardening products you use; the building you work in; the home you live in; and the water you drink. Getting rid of toxicity on all fronts is crucial to fighting inflammation. Doing periodic cleanses of your organs of elimination can make a huge difference in bringing inflammation down. You can take my "How Toxic Are You?" quiz at http://www.juiceladycherie .com/Juice/toxic-take-the-quiz/. If you have a high score, it's very important that you cleanse your body. Get my book *Juicing, Fasting, and Detoxing for Life*. Start with the colon cleanse, then liver/gallbladder, kidney/bladder, lung, lymphatic system, and skin and blood. You will find cleanse kits on my website to assist in your cleansing process.

Leaky gut syndrome

When your cortisol is elevated due to stress or your thyroid and adrenal hormone levels fluctuate due to stress or burning the midnight oil, your intestinal lining becomes more permeable. When you eat during this time, partially undigested food, toxins, viruses, yeast, and bacteria have the opportunity to pass through the intestinal wall and access the bloodstream. This is leaky gut syndrome. When the intestinal lining is repeatedly damaged due to stress hormones and/or a pro-inflammatory diet, damaged cells are unable to do their job well. The intestines are unable to properly absorb nutrients and enzymes that are vital to proper digestion. Eventually digestion is impaired and absorption of nutrients is affected. As this scenario progresses, your body initiates an attack on foreign invaders. It responds with inflammation, allergic reactions, and various symptoms related to a variety of diseases. It can even turn on itself, and the person is diagnosed with an autoimmune disease.

Inactivity

Lack of exercise can directly lead to low-grade inflammation. According to Western Washington University, "Skeletal muscles act as an endocrine organ by influencing metabolism and modifying immune system message production in other tissues including endothelial and adipose tissues. As skeletal muscles perform work, they produce and release anti-inflammatory substances into the blood."[5] When you are active, markers of inflammation such as C-reactive protein are reduced. If you sit at a desk for a good portion of the day, it is important to get up and move around as much as possible. Stand up when you talk on the phone. Do some knee bends or stretches when you take a break. Walk on your lunch hour. Walk after dinner. Park your car a little farther away than usual so you can walk a few more steps. Ride your stationary bike while you talk on the phone or watch the evening news. Get a gym membership, and work out three times a week. Continually think of ways to get more movement into your life.

Obesity

Fat cells may actually play a role in promoting inflammation. Low-grade inflammation of adipose (fat) tissue can result from chronic activation of the innate immune system. Research has shown an association between inflammatory cytokines and proteins and adipose tissue function.[6] Obese individuals have higher levels of C-reactive protein.[7]

POST-MENOPAUSAL WOMEN, HORMONE REPLACEMENT THERAPY (HRT), AND VASCULAR INFLAMMATION

Hormone replacement therapy (HRT) has a vascular inflammation effect and may lead to increased risk of cardiovascular disease.[8] Data from the Women's Health Initiative showed that elevated levels of C-reactive protein and interleukin-6 (IL-6) is both pro-inflammatory and anti-inflammatory. When out of balance, it stimulates inflammatory and disease processes. Both elevated CRP and IL-6 were associated with HRT use, but not as significant in women who exercised while taking hormone replacement therapy (HRT). C-reactive protein levels were significantly higher in sedentary HRT users.[9] This study provides evidence that exercise may be beneficial to counteract the negative impacts of HRT. However, it is far better to use plant hormones and also to exercise.

Eating a pro-inflammatory diet

Our Western diet, loaded with refined foods, sugars, additives, and fillers, contributes to inflammation especially in the cells of the blood vessel walls as well as throughout the entire body. The next two chapters are devoted to the anti-inflammatory diet because many health professionals believe that our modern diet is the number one contributor to inflammation.

Chapter 2

FOODS AND FACTORS THAT CONTRIBUTE TO INFLAMMATION

*Health is like money, we never have a true
idea of its value until we lose it.*[1]
—JOSH BILLINGS

W E'VE SLIPPED INTO a destructive cycle eating the standard American diet, which places an emphasis on foods that directly contribute to inflammation. This diet causes the production of cortisol and contributes to elevated stress levels. The main staples of a typical American diet—sugar, starch, corn, soy, and grains (gluten)—are undoubtedly the biggest contributors to chronic inflammation. From breakfast to dinner Americans serve up foods that stoke the inflammatory fire in the body. Following are the foods you should avoid to get inflammation under control and enjoy vibrant health.

Shun Sugar and Artificial and Low-Cal Sweeteners

America loves its sugar. Most of us are sugar babies; we've been raised on this stuff. From snacks and soft drinks to breakfast cereals and desserts, we just can't get enough of it. But the sweet side has a downside. Our addiction to sweets is slowly killing us. We're seduced with added sugar in processed foods, sauces, dressings, snacks, and beverages. This is doubling our chances of heart-related premature death, cancer, diabetes, and obesity.

Sugar and other foods with high-glycemic value spike insulin levels and place the immune system on high alert. When blood sugar spikes, we crave more sweets, starch, refined flour goods, salt, and junk food. In response to an inflammatory diet, the body produces more cortisol, which causes further inflammation, more cortisol production, higher insulin levels, more cravings—and on and on it goes in an unending cycle.

As a result, high insulin levels activate enzymes that raise levels of arachidonic acid in our blood. Arachidonic acid is a natural fatty acid found in certain foods and is also made in the body. It is essential to life in small amounts, but it is also the building block of inflammatory hormones. We do not want it in abundance.

Consuming large amounts of sugar, fructose, artificial sweeteners, and low-calorie sweeteners such as sugar alcohols cause your gut bacteria to adapt in a way that interferes with your satiety signals and metabolism, according to a paper published in *Obesity Reviews*.[2] The sweetener-adapted bacteria thrive and become more efficient at processing large amounts of sugars, and they produce more and more short-chain fatty acids. The short-chain fatty acids promote inflammation in the lining of the gut.

A study in healthy, middle-aged women showed that high glycemic loads were related to high levels of C-reactive protein, independent of weight and total caloric intake.[3]

Sometimes inflammation can be present and you will not even know it's there. This type of chronic, low-grade inflammation is known as silent inflammation, and we know from studies that excess sugar intake is associated with the silent type.

To break this cycle, it's imperative to avoid sugar, fructose, artificial sweeteners, low-calorie sweeteners, corn syrup, dextrose, pancake syrup, maltose, sorghum, and sucrose. Many people are addicted to sweeteners, so it takes some effort to avoid sweets. Take heart. After about two weeks the cravings go away.

Here's what to avoid:

- Boxed cereals and breakfast bars
- Coffee drinks with sweetened syrup
- Commercially made foods with added sweeteners; read the labels
- Energy bars
- Pastries, cupcakes, desserts, candies
- Protein powders with added sugars
- Snacks and junk food
- Soft drinks, fruit drinks, punch (one Coke is equal to eating about ten sugar cubes)

THE SKINNY ON DIET SODAS

Artificial sweeteners are hundreds to thousands of times sweeter than regular sugar, activating a person's preference for more sweet foods over any other substance. They trick your metabolism into thinking sugar is being consumed. This prompts your body to pump out insulin, the fat storage hormone, which promotes belly fat that sticks around like caramel on an apple.

It also confuses and slows your metabolism; you will burn fewer calories. It makes you hungrier, and you crave even more sugar and starch such as bread and pasta. In animal studies rats that consumed more artificial sweeteners ate more, their metabolism slowed down, and they gained 14 percent more body fat in just two weeks, even though they ate fewer calories. In population studies there was a 200 percent increased risk of obesity in diet soda drinkers.[4]

Say No to Refined Grains

Refined grains are devoid of fiber and vitamin B and loaded with starch. This makes them similar to refined sugars—both are empty calories.

Like refined sugars, they also have a higher glycemic index than unprocessed grains. When consistently consumed, they can hasten the onset of inflammation and degenerative diseases such as cancer, coronary heart disease, and diabetes.

Wipe Out Wheat

The main problem with wheat is gluten. Gliadins, components of gluten are proteins found in wheat (durum, emmer, spelt, farina, farro, and kamut), rye, barley, and triticale; they are responsible for the elastic texture of dough. Starting in the 1960s, we have been manipulating wheat to obtain fluffier bread. Some varieties of wheat contain more gluten, so that's what they manipulate to get more gluten. *Gluten* comes from the Latin word for glue. Its adhesive properties hold bread together. However, this glue interferes with the breakdown and absorption of nutrients, including the nutrients from other foods in the same meal. As a result we get a "glued-together," constipating mix in the gut rather than a nutritious, easily digested meal. The undigested gluten then triggers the immune system to attack the lining of the small intestine and causes symptoms such as diarrhea, constipation, nausea, bloating, and abdominal pain. It can lead to serious problems for some people, such as celiac disease.

We eat far too much gluten today. Just take a look at the typical American diet—a bagel or toast for breakfast, a sandwich or hamburger for lunch, and rolls, pizza, or pasta for dinner. That's a lot of grain (and gluten) in just one day. Even larger amounts are consumed if we take into consideration common snacks such as crackers and chips made with grains, and desserts such as cookies and cakes. Additionally, commercial grain-based products that line grocery store shelves and are served at restaurants such as breading and fillers are commonplace. These products produce mucus, raise blood sugar levels, and increase inflammation. Plus, breads are often filled with ingredients that are not food, such as the chemical azodicarbonamide that is also used in yoga mats, synthetic leather, and shoe rubber, along with dough conditioners potassium bromade (interferes with iodine absorption), artificial flavorings or coloring,

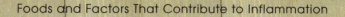

genetically modified organisms (GMOs), and L-cysteine, an amino acid that extends shelf life and is often made from human hair gathered off the floors of Chinese hair salons.

Gluten and thyroid inflammation

Although there is some research linking celiac disease and Hashimoto's disease, the impact gluten has on thyroid function still isn't widely accepted as fact. However, an increasing number of medical professionals are sharing their expertise and success using a gluten-free diet to alleviate some of the symptoms of thyroid imbalances. According to Dr. Datis Kharrazian, "Because the molecular structure of gluten so closely resembles that of the thyroid gland, the problem may be one of mistaken identity. Every time undigested gluten mistakenly slips into the bloodstream, the immune system responds by destroying it for removal."[5] Over time the body goes haywire. Because the molecular structure of gluten so closely resembles that of the thyroid, the body starts to attack the thyroid—a case of mistaken identity. Once the attack is set in motion, there's no way to turn it off. A person with Hashimoto's autoimmune thyroid must be on a gluten-free diet. If you eat gluten, it can affect you for up to six months. People with low thyroid also greatly benefit from a gluten-free diet.[6]

Those with thyroid conditions often ask about goitrogenic foods (which means iodine blockers) that include soy, peanuts, millet, and cruciferous vegetables: broccoli, brussels sprouts, cauliflower, cabbage, and kale. These marvelous vegetables are not on the list of foods that contribute to inflammation; rather, they fight inflammation, cancer, and a host of ailments. But they are on the avoid list for those with hypothyroid or Hashimoto's thyroiditis. You may be able to include them raw (some can; some can't), but not every day. Mostly you should cook, lightly steam, or ferment them, which deactivates the glucosinolates, thus diminishing their goitrogneic activity.

It is always best to rotate your greens. Dr. Craig Maxwell encourages his patients with thyroid issues to include cruciferous vegetables. He says, "In my experience, the lab values (TSH, Free T3, and Free

T4) used to evaluate thyroid function have remained in the same range whether patients eat them or not."[7] If you have thyroid problems, you should definitely avoid the other goitrogenic foods: peanuts and peanut butter, millet, and all soy products (soy blocks the activity of the TPO enzyme). Canola oil (rapeseed) is also a goitrogen and should be eliminated. It is highly processed and made from genetically modified crops as well.

Refuse Refined Table Salt

Table salt is a manufactured form of sodium called sodium chloride. It is a highly refined, man-made substance produced by taking either natural salt or crude oil flake leftovers and cooking it at 1,200 degrees Fahrenheit. Once the salt is heated to this temperature, it loses the majority of the minerals. Then they add iodine and harmful chemicals such as:

- Anti-caking agents
- Bleach
- Fluoride
- Monosodium glutamate (MSG)
- Potassium iodide
- Solo-Co-aluminate and other aluminum derivatives

These additives and food preservatives can contribute to serious health problems. This salt is also highly acidic, which can contribute to chronic inflammation. You should use only natural sea salt, gray salt, or pink Himalayan salt.

Forget Feedlot-Raised Meats

Commercially raised animals are fed mostly grains, soybeans, and corn—a diet that is high in pro-inflammatory omega-6 fatty acids and low in anti-inflammatory omega-3 fats. Omega-6 fatty acids are pro-inflammatory because they are broken down by the body and converted into prostaglandins and other inflammatory proteins. These proteins cause inflammation. They are kept in crowded living conditions where they gain excess weight. This results in highly saturated fat. To force them to grow faster and prevent them from getting sick, they are injected with hormones and antibiotics. Animal foods including beef, lamb, poultry, and eggs have been safely eaten for thousands of years without causing problems. Modern-day diseases associated with the Western diet include eating large quantities of cheap feedlot-raised meat that is high in arachidonic acid, an omega-6 fat that can trigger joint pain and inflammation. The same goes for chickens and eggs raised in cages or close quarters with conventional food. Most of the animal products in the supermarkets and restaurants come from feedlot farms. Completely avoid them.

Steer Away From Unhealthy Oils

Eliminate all hydrogenated and partially hydrogenated oils, trans fats, and polyunsaturated vegetable oils, including safflower, sunflower, corn, and soy along with canola oil (a big GMO crop). The American diet is loaded with omega-6 oils and deficient in the anti-inflammatory omega-3 oils found in vegetables; seeds like flax, hemp, and chia; and walnuts, plus fatty cold-water fish. Too much omega-6 from refined vegetable oils results in inflammatory chemicals circulating in the body, which reduce the ability of our cells to function normally. Also, polyunsaturated oils oxidize easily, meaning they react with oxygen and form an oxide. When heated, vegetable oils can oxidize quickly and cause free-radical damage; at high heat they form trans fats that generate even more free radicals, which can damage healthy cells, trigger inflammation, and LDL (bad cholesterol) levels. Partially hydrogenated oils, such as in margarine, are equally as damaging.

The unhealthy oils are in most salad dressings, mayonnaise, packaged foods, and convenience foods. When you eat out, your food will most likely be prepared with these oils, unless you eat in a health-oriented restaurant or you order food that is grilled and get olive oil and vinegar for your salad.

Ditch the Dairy

Dairy (and wheat) are among the most irritating foods for our systems since they encourage the production of mucus (phlegm) in the body. In Chinese medicine it's known as "dampness." Mucus leads to inflammation and a host of common symptoms such as low energy, poor sleep, and impaired digestion. Dairy is also a common allergen that can trigger inflammatory responses such as stomach distress, constipation, diarrhea, skin rashes, acne, hives, and breathing difficulties in susceptible people. Dr. David Ludwig and Dr. Walter Willett from Harvard (published in the *Journal of the American Medical Association*) found no data to support the claim that the consumption of dairy leads to better bones, weight loss, or improved health. They also found some serious risks tied to dairy consumption, including weight gain, increased cancer risk, and increased fracture risk. It turns out milk does not build strong bones! They also found that dairy may cause other problems such as constipation, irritable bowel syndrome, bloating, gas, diarrhea, allergies, eczema, and acne.[8]

Curb Caffeine Intake

A study published in 2004 in the *American Journal of Clinical Nutrition* found a relationship between moderate to high coffee consumption and increased inflammation, in both men and women who drank coffee. Interleukin-6 and C-reactive protein (inflammation markers) were significantly higher than with non-coffee drinkers. This relationship could explain, in part, the negative effect of increased coffee intake on the cardiovascular system.[9] Note that caffeine is also found in black tea and soda (an even more inflammatory beverage than coffee).

Beware of the Buzz on Alcohol

Beer, hard cider, liquor, liqueur, and wine promote inflammation. Regular consumption of alcohol has been known to cause irritation and inflammation of the esophagus, larynx, and liver. Overconsumption of alcohol can increase the body's inflammatory response from head to toe. Chronic inflammation promotes tumor growth and cancer at the sites of repeated irritation. According to Dr. Mark Hyman, you should take a six- to eight-week break from alcohol; then don't reintegrate drinking every day. He says two to three servings of alcohol is the maximum you should ingest per week. A serving size is:

- 12 fluid ounces beer
- 4- to 5-fluid-ounce glass wine (choose organic; grapes are heavily sprayed)
- 1.5 fluid ounces spirits

If you drink more than this in a week you are exposing yourself to serious health risks including dementia, depression, and an increased risk of type 2 diabetes that can contribute to a wide variety of health conditions including high blood pressure and heart disease.[10]

Avoid Irradiated Food

Food irradiation has been taking place in conventional vegetables, meats, and other nonorganic products for years. It kills insects and other bugs that may have crawled into foods before being shipped to the grocery store. Conventionally grown produce, from apples to zucchini, is routinely irradiated. At first it may seem that food irradiation to kill bacteria and bugs on conventional vegetables and meat should be common practice. After all, spinach irradiated to kill salmonella is happy spinach, right? Not necessarily.

Food irradiation involves exposing food to high levels of radiation to kill insects, bacteria, fungus, and mold, and to give food a longer shelf life. Although the idea of radiating food sounds quite unappetizing, it has been practiced in the United States since the 1960s, when the FDA approved irradiation of wheat and white potatoes. (Currently the eyes of white potatoes are painted with chemicals to keep them from sprouting.)

During the 1980s they approved irradiation of spices and seasonings, pork, fresh fruit, and dried and dehydrated substances. Poultry received approval for irradiation in 1990 and red meat in 1997.

Purchase only organic produce. The only good thing is that in the United States, food growers and manufacturers are supposed to label food that is irradiated, so avoidance of irradiated foods is possible if one shops carefully. Since 1986 all irradiated products must carry the international symbol called a radura, which is a flower within a circle and is similar to the symbol for the Environmental Protection Agency. However, I have not seen a radura symbol yet on any produce where I shop.

Say No to GMO

What do tortilla chips, soy milk, and canola oil have in common? They are all made from the top GMO crops in North America. About 85 percent of the corn grown in the US is genetically engineered to either produce an insecticide or to survive the application of herbicide. And about 91 to 93 percent of all soybeans are genetically engineered to survive massive doses of Roundup herbicide.[11]

Many of these products you would not want anyway, but when it comes to certain vegetables, unless you buy organically grown, it's quite probable you'll be eating genetically modified food. And that should cause you great concern. We are the human "guinea pigs" when it comes to genetically modified (GM) foods. Studies with rats have shown that GM foods promote tumors and indicate that we should be very concerned about eating GM foods. A French study—the most comprehensive GMO safety assessment ever conducted—highlights that concern. It involved two hundred rats and spanned two years, the life expectancy of the species of rat used. The researchers say their results show "severe adverse health effects, including mammary tumors and kidney and liver damage, leading to premature death" from Roundup-Ready corn and Roundup herbicide.[12]

Some estimates say that as many as thirty thousand different products on grocery store shelves are genetically modified, which is largely because many processed foods contain some form of soy or corn.

When trying to avoid these top GM crops, you'll need to watch out for maltodextrin, soy lecithin, soy oil, textured vegetable protein (soy), canola oil, corn products, and high fructose corn syrup. Other GM crops to avoid include some varieties of zucchini, crookneck squash, papayas from Hawaii, milk containing rbGH, rennet (containing genetically modified enzymes) used to make hard cheeses, and aspartame (NutraSweet).

Move on From Microwaved Food

Cooking in a microwave oven is not recommend as it creates toxic by-products such as d-Nitrosodiethanolamine (a well-known cancer-causing agent) in the food cooked. It also causes alteration in the breakdown of glucoside and galactoside elements within frozen fruits when thawed in a microwave oven, and cancer-causing free radicals were formed within certain trace-mineral molecular formations in plants, especially in raw root vegetables. I (Cherie) don't even use a microwave to heat water; it's that destructive. Such water can kill plants.

Unlikely Culprits That Contribute to Inflammation

Nightshade vegetables

The link between the nightshade family, chronic pain, and inflammation is not well known by many people. Although not true for everyone, this family of foods is thought to cause inflammation and arthritis symptoms in about 30 percent of the population. Nightshades belong to the Solanaceae family, which sport some of the most popular foods we consume, such as tomatoes, potatoes, all types of peppers (both hot and bell peppers; not black pepper or peppercorns), and eggplant. Although not truly nightshades, blueberries, huckleberries, goji berries, and ashwaganda share the same alkaloids. However, they are not problematic for most people. The glycoalkaloids in potatoes are known to contribute to irritable bowel syndrome (IBS) and negatively affect intestinal permeability. According to Dr. Marvin Childers, "When these inhibitors accumulate in the body, alone or with other cholinesterase inhibitors such as caffeine or food impurities containing systemic cholinesterase inhibiting pesticides, the result may be a paralytic-like muscle spasm, aches, pains, tenderness, inflammation, and stiff body movements."[13]

Many people who suffer with arthritis or an arthritis-related disease such as lupus, rheumatism, and other musculoskeletal pain disorders have discovered that consuming foods from the nightshade family is a major factor in their poor health.

The best way to determine if you are sensitive to the nightshade family is to do the nightshade elimination and challenge. This is similar to the elimination diet. You omit all nightshade foods for three months. You should read labels and look for anything such as potato starch or a form of one of these foods. Also be aware they can show up in over-the-counter or prescription medications. After three months you will introduce one nightshade food at a time. If you experience aches, pains, stiffness, loss of energy, headaches, or respiratory problems, you may be sensitive to this family of foods. Be aware that you could get a delayed reaction a couple of days later; not everyone reacts immediately after ingesting certain foods. Also, note that soy sauce made in America is usually made with genetically modified (GMO) soy beans, which are cut with the nightshade plant petunia.

Citrus: not for some

Most people are not sensitive to citrus fruits. However, for those who have a citrus sensitivity, these fruits can cause inflammation and contribute to the development of stiffness, arthritis, and chronic diseases. If citrus sensitivity affects you, try tart cherries instead, which have the highest anti-inflammatory content of any food, according to research from the Oregon Health and Science University.[14]

Food allergens

Food allergens can cause and/or contribute to the inflammatory process throughout the body. Common allergens like casein (in dairy) and gluten (in wheat, barley, rye, spelt, and oats) can spark the inflammatory cascade. Everyone who suffers from celiac disease knows about inflammation in the gut caused by gluten. When a person eats foods they are sensitive to, their heart rate will rise sixteen beats per minute or more. There is an app that has been developed to help you detect food sensitivities by measuring your pulse in the morning and then before and after you eat. This is the latest technology in food sensitivity detection from SweetWater Health.[15]

Chapter 3

CHANGE YOUR DIET; CHANGE YOUR LIFE!

Let food be thy medicine and medicine be thy food.[1]
—HIPPOCRATES

I HAVE HELPED THOUSANDS of people from all over the world with their heath and nutrition. When they've been willing to change their diet and to juice each day, their health and indeed their entire lives have changed. Inflammation is controlled. Aches and pains disappear like mist in the morning sun. All sorts of ailments are healed. They enjoy energy to do many things they could never do before.

As you learned in the introduction, juicing and a healthy, whole-foods diet changed my life. I had suffered with chronic fatigue syndrome and fibromyalgia for several years until it progressed to the point where I could no longer work. I searched for answers because no one in the medical profession could help me. That's when I discovered juicing and the power of a whole-foods, anti-inflammatory diet. I cut out everything that wasn't a life-giving food and drank about a quart of fresh veggie juice a day.

Within three months all my pain, fatigue, brain fog, and flu-like symptoms were gone. I felt like a brand-new person.

DIET CHANGES GAVE HER A NEW LIFE

I've come a long way from being told I am prediabetic and have high cholesterol. I had been struggling to go up a short flight of stairs. Now I am enjoying life. I hike, dance the night away, rock climb, skate, and water ski. This is all because of changing my eating habits and juicing.

—Iris

The modern diet offers us an inverted ratio of fatty acids (omega-3, -6, and -9), too much sugar and carbs, and an abundance of wheat, dairy, soy, corn, and other common allergenic, inflammatory foods. "What you eat and how much you exercise are the most important factors governing inflammation," says Mark Hyman, MD.[2] Most of the factors for ridding yourself of inflammation lie within your control. You have the power to change and heal your body. It starts with what you choose to eat each day.

Choose Real, Whole Food

Often we hear the term *real foods* or *whole foods*, which is meant to counter substances that are man-made—whipped up in factories and spun out in forms that are anything but real or whole. These foods have become the basis of the American diet, but they should not be called food. They are processed and depleted of natural nutrients and filled with chemicals to promote longer shelf life, ease of transportation, and longer storage. They are designed with one thing in mind—flavor you'll like and the right substances to get you addicted to that product. Despite a variety of flavors, textures, and shapes, most of these products are manufactured from the same mono-cultured crops—wheat, corn, soy, and potatoes. They are depleted in nutrients due to growth in high-density environments and depleted soils, while also being saturated with petroleum-based fertilizers. They are among the biggest GMO crops in America. Due to this stressful growth situation, they are susceptible to pests. Commercial agriculture deals with their susceptibility by spraying them with high amounts of insecticides or by producing GMO "franken-plants" that have pesticides built right into the plant, such as Monsanto's Roundup Ready alfalfa and corn. This poses alarming threats to our health, our ecosystem, and our long-term food supply.

Plant nutrient values are further diminished in the course of processing and storage, so the processed foods are fortified with synthetic vitamins and minerals. Flavorings are added to improve the taste because they have very little flavor left. These foods are addictive, carcinogenic, and inflammatory, while being void of nutrients necessary for cellular function. They deliver empty calories that get stored as fat because the body can't use them for most of its functions.

Real foods are the foods that are the least processed. They are closest to their natural form and, therefore, retain the most nutrient value and deliver the highest health benefits. They are rich in flavor. They retain natural diversity of tastes. They have high nutrient and antioxidant content. And, if they are organically grown, seasonal, and local foods, they are the healthiest choices possible.

A Miracle Before Our Eyes

In 1991 Lois was diagnosed with rheumatoid arthritis (RA) by the Mayo Clinic. She was healed not long after. In 1992 she and her husband returned to the mission field where they worked until April 2011. They had flown to Poland and were waiting for a van at 11:30 p.m. when her husband had a heart attack. He died right there on the sidewalk of a foreign street. Lois was in shock. She said it felt like a bad dream. She had to wait eight days in Poland before she could bring his body home.

After this trauma her RA returned. By the summer of 2013 she suffered from crippling RA and was bedridden, only able to use a wheelchair or walker occasionally. She prayed and prayed for healing, but her disease progressed. In early March of 2014 she received a very discouraging medical diagnosis—her swelling and blood infection was high. Right after that, she saw *It's Supernatural!*, where I was interviewed by Sid Roth. That show gave her hope. Her daughter, Rudina, visited my website and found out about our retreat.

Lois arrived in a great deal of pain with very swollen feet from sitting for many hours in the car driving from Chicago to Glorieta, New Mexico. She had a difficult time walking into the buildings. But things began to change for her rather quickly. The anti-inflammatory diet of vegetable juices, green smoothies, and raw foods changed her physiology. The pain started to lessen. My husband's emotional and mental detox classes helped her identify the grief, shock, and trauma that had adversely affected her body with toxic chemicals the emotions produce. Wednesday evening offered her an opportunity to let go of those emotions in our Taize service. Prayer in the mornings fed her spirit.

Wednesday evening back in their room, just four days after arriving, Lois told her daughter she thought she could walk and showed Rudina that she could take steps without her walker. By Thursday she was standing up straight. Rudina had often told her mom to stand up straight, but she couldn't because the pain was too intense. Thursday afternoon she felt she just had to tell me what had happened, but I was always surrounded by people. Then suddenly everyone left the lecture room and we were there alone.

She said, "Cherie, I have something I want to show you." Her daughter pushed aside some chairs—and Lois started walking across the floor without assistance. What a miracle! When she and Rudina walked into the dining hall, she was pushing her walker in front of her and then walked without it. The whole room burst into cheers and tears!

Lois isn't unique. You can find healing and abundant health too. Here's what you can choose to promote your anti-inflammatory, vibrant health program.

Vegetables, Fruit, Sprouts, and Vegetable Juices

These are your most alkalizing foods; they are also super anti-inflammatory. Your goal is to balance the pH level of your body. For good health and keeping inflammation in control, our bodies need to be slightly alkaline with a pH between 7.35 and 7.45. Sounds rather simple right? Well, this is not regular mathematics based on arithmetic; pH operates on a logarithmic scale in multiples of ten. A unit decrease in pH means a tenfold increase in acid. For example, the difference between a food rated four and one rated five means the four is ten times more acidic. The majority of the foods eaten in America are acid forming in their final breakdown in the body. These foods include meat, poultry, fish, dairy, grains, some legumes, sugar, coffee, black tea, soda, alcohol, and junk food. The alkaline-based foods are vegetables, fruit, juices, sprouts, grasses such as wheatgrass and barley grass, seeds (quinoa is a seed), and nuts. As you can see, typical American foods are focused mainly on the acid-forming foods.

The best way to neutralize acids in the body is through the food we eat. Because it requires a delicate balance, we need to eat a very alkaline-rich diet to achieve this balance and promote good health. Fruits and vegetables are our best friends when it comes to alkalinity. They contain powerful antioxidants to boost the immune system and prevent chronic inflammation. Also, fruits and vegetables are high in antioxidants and phytonutrients such as bioflavonoids, which improve blood vessel strength and reduce the tendency of capillaries to leak fluid. To shift the body in the direction of alkaline balance, make alkaline foods about 75 percent of your diet. To help you reach this goal, we've included plenty of delicious juice, smoothie, and vegetable recipes in the anti-inflammation diet.

Here's what you should emphasize.

Vegetables and fruit—rich in antioxidants

Antioxidants are compounds found especially in brightly colored vegetables and fruit. They include vitamins A, C, and E; glutathione;

beta-carotene; lycopene; coenzyme Q_{10}; and the trace mineral selenium. A 2009 study with humans and mice demonstrated that antioxidants reduce inflammation.[3]

How many servings of vegetables and fruit should you eat?

The study based on the Health Survey for England found that people who ate seven or more portions per day of fruit and vegetables had a 42 percent lower chance of dying prematurely.[4] When researchers combined findings from the Harvard studies with several other long-term studies in the United States and Europe, and looked at coronary heart disease and stroke separately, they found a similar protective effect: individuals who ate more than five servings of fruits and vegetables per had roughly a 20 percent lower risk of coronary heart disease and stroke, compared with individuals who ate less than three servings per day.[5]

- Green smoothies. Depending on the amount of greens and fruit, this could add up to one to two servings

- Organic fruits and vegetables. Eat six to nine servings a day (a serving is one-half cup cooked and one cup raw).

- Vegetable juices. Drink one to three glasses of freshly made vegetable juice each day. This can significantly help in alkalizing your body and provides an abundance of antioxidants to bind up free radicals. Juicing is the single most important thing you can do to quell inflammation. (One-half cup of juice equals a serving.) A 2006 Vanderbilt University study found that people who consumed three or more servings of fruit and vegetable juices each week appeared to be 76 percent less likely to develop signs of Alzheimer's over ten years than those who drank fewer than one serving a week.[6]

Antioxidant Power Smoothie

Berries help prevent damaging effects of free radicals and inflammation by turning off the inflammation signals triggered by cytokines and COX-2s, making them an ideal part of your diet.

1 cup unsweetened plant milk such as hemp, coconut, or almond milk
½ cup blueberries
1 pear
½ cup baby spinach
1 tsp. Indian gooseberry extract (optional)*
1 Tbsp. flaxseed
Ice cubes (optional, depending on how cold you like your smoothie)

Add all the ingredients to a blender and process until smooth.
    *At 3277 umol TE/100g, gooseberries have oxygen radical absorbance capacity (ORAC) value comparable to that of red currants (3387 umol TE/100g)—among the highest ORAC value.

Black cherries for joint pain and arthritis

Tart cherries may help reduce chronic inflammation, especially for people suffering from joint pain and arthritis, according to research. The researchers suggest tart cherries have the "highest anti-inflammatory content of any food" and can help people with osteoarthritis manage their disease. A study from University of California at Davis found that regular consumption of cherries for twenty-eight days produced a decrease in biochemical signs of inflammation in blood, including a 25 percent reduction in C-reactive protein (CRP), the most widely studied marker of inflammation. Elevation of CRP in blood is associated with an increased risk of heart disease and stroke.[7]

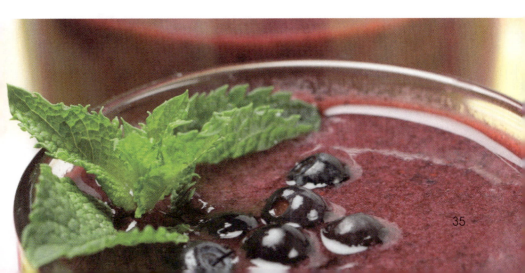

Chocolate Cherry Shake

1 Tbsp. unsweetened, unprocessed cocoa powder
½ cup frozen dark cherries, pitted
1 cup coconut, almond, or flax milk
½ tsp. pure vanilla extract
Several drops of liquid stevia (suggest Sweet Leaf Vanilla Crème)
Ice cubes as desired

Place all ingredients in a blender and process until smooth.

Seeds and nuts

Raw nuts and seeds, especially almonds, walnuts, cashews, sunflower, flax, sesame, and pumpkin seeds, are a rich source of lignans. Lignans are unique fiber-related polyphenols that provide us with antioxidant benefits, fiber-like benefits, and also act as phytoestrogens.

Among all commonly eaten foods, researchers rank flaxseeds as the number one source of lignans. Flaxseeds contain a combination of omega-3 fatty acids, high-lignan content, and mucilage gums, which make them a superior anti-inflammatory food.

Wild foods

Wild foods like dandelion greens, nettles, chickweed, wood sorrel, wild salad greens, and shepherd's purse offer us nutrients found nowhere else in nature. Since people have adapted to eating wild plants for several hundred thousand years, problems will arise when we try to eat hybridized and genetically engineered fruits and veggies. Our physiology is not programmed to handle this. Include more wild foods in your diet, which send the ancient message of life to your hungry cells.

Sweet Wild Smoothie

1 pear, Bartlett or Asian
½ green apple
1 large handful dandelion greens* or other wild greens
1 cup coconut milk
Juice of ½ lemon
¼ cup flaxseeds
1 tsp. turmeric
6 ice cubes (optional)

Place all ingredients in a blender and process until a creamy smoothie. Serves 2.

*Dandelion has been used as a traditional remedy to treat liver problems, infections, swelling, water retention, breast problems, gallbladder problems, pneumonia, and viruses. Studies have shown it stimulates bile flow and has a mild diuretic effect.

Veggies That Have Special Anti-Inflammatory Properties

- Asparagus contains saponins—phytonutrients that have repeatedly been shown to have anti-inflammatory and anticancer properties. Its intake has also been associated with improved blood pressure, blood sugar regulation, and better control of blood fat levels. It is also a natural diuretic.

- Beets contain phytonutrients called betalains. Betanin and vulgaxanthin are the two most-studied betalains from beets. Each has been shown to provide antioxidant, anti-inflammatory, and detoxification effects. Beets have also been shown to lower blood pressure.

JANET'S PAIN IS GONE

I know for sure that the juices have healed my arthritis and tennis elbow. Also, my finger joints were very swollen, and now they are normal as are my husband's. My husband has taken no medication since his heart attack. My friend has been healed of her pain too. A GP I know is very interested now. I think the beetroot juice is so healing. Cherie, it's just amazing. I know God has given us these foods for sure. It's so exciting.

- Carrot has anti-inflammatory properties and provides anti-inflammatory benefits that were significant even when compared to anti-inflammatory drugs like aspirin, ibuprofen, naproxen, and Celebrex.

- Celery is a good source of vitamin C, beta-carotene, sodium, and manganese—phenolic antioxidants that have been shown to reduce inflammation. If you are suffering from joint pains, lung infections, asthma, or acne, eating and juicing more celery will bring much-needed relief. It also helps you calm down and relieves stress. The minerals in celery, especially magnesium, soothe the nervous system. If you enjoy celery in the evening, you may sleep better. Also, celery juice may lower your blood pressure. A twenty-year animal study found that 3-n-butylphthalide, an extract found in celery, lowers blood pressure and cholesterol levels. The daily dose needed to gain this benefit appeared to be about four stalks, which explains why one might want to get it through juice.[8]

- Fennel is rich in the phytonutrient anethole. This nutrient has repeatedly been shown to reduce inflammation and to help prevent the occurrence of cancer.

- Kale. Research has identified more than forty-five different flavonoids in kale. With kaempferol and quercetin at the top of the list, kale's flavonoids and antioxidants have anti-inflammatory benefits that help quell chronic inflammation and oxidative stress.

- Spinach. Glycoglycerolipid, a nutrient in spinach, can help protect the lining of the digestive tract especially from damage related to inflammation.

Anti-Inflammatory Fruit

- Avocados contain very important fats, namely the phytosterols, which account for a major portion of their fat. The fats in avocado are key supporters of our inflammatory system and help keep inflammation under control.

- Berries contain antioxidants that can help your body fight oxidative stress caused by free radicals. Berries contain polyphenol compounds shown to have anti-inflammatory activity in humans. Among the most notable polyphenols in berries are anthocyanins, responsible for their distinctive colors of red, blue, and purple. Berries have been studied widely for their antioxidant properties; data suggest important effects on inflammatory pathways.[9] Eating a diet rich in antioxidants can help to protect your skin and hair and fight inflammation.

- Papaya has several unique protein-digesting enzymes, including papain and chymopapain, which have been shown to help lower inflammation.

- Peaches contain phenolic compounds that prevent the oxidization of low-density lipoprotein (LDL) cholesterol. (It is oxidized LDL (oxLDL) that is dangerous; most blood tests don't distinguish this from non-oxidized LDL.) These phenolic compounds can help fight inflammation associated with metabolic syndrome—a combination of medical disorders that increases the risk of obesity, type 2 diabetes, and cardiovascular disease.

- Pears contain phytonutrients that have been shown to provide anti-inflammatory benefits. They have been associated with decreased risk of several common diseases associated with chronic inflammation and excessive oxidative stress.

The Incredible Benefits of Omega-3 Fatty Acids

Omega-3s are essential fatty acids that help reduce inflammation throughout your body, including your brain. An inappropriate balance of fatty acids (too much omega-6; too little omega-3) contributes to the development of inflammation and disease, while a proper balance helps keep inflammation under control and improves health. A healthy diet should consist of roughly two to four times more omega-3 fatty acids than omega-6 fats. The typical American diet tends to contain fourteen to twenty-five times more omega-6 fats. Many researchers believe this imbalance is a significant factor in the rising rate of inflammatory disorders in the United States.

To increase your omega-3 fats, choose wild trout and wild-caught Alaskan salmon, which is regularly tested and found to have no significant level of Fukushima radiation. (You should avoid other fish at this time due to radiation pollution.) Also include krill oil, cod liver oil, flax, hemp, chia seeds, and walnuts.

Use Only Healthy Oils

Myocardial infarction (MI) was almost nonexistent in 1910 and caused no more than 3,000 deaths per year in 1930. By 1960, there were at least 500,000 MI deaths per year in the U.S. What lifestyle changes had caused this increase? One of the major changes in this country was the mainstream introduction of polyunsaturated cooking oils in the 1940s. Until World War II they were not popularly used. But when ships couldn't transport coconut oil from Asia and the South Pacific due to the war, the vegetable oil industry stepped up production.[10]

There is a correlation between polyunsaturated cooking oils, the rise of heart disease, and oxidized LDL (oxLDL), which is formed when the lipids in LDL particles react with oxygen and break down. This happens specifically to the unsaturated fats in LDL, because saturated fats, by their chemical nature, are very resistant to oxidative damage. Polyunsaturated fats are much more susceptible to oxidative damage than saturated or monounsaturated fats. Linoleic acid (the omega-6 fatty acid found abundantly in industrial seed oils) is the main polyunsaturated fatty acid in LDL.[11]

It is imperative to avoid safflower, sunflower, soy, corn, and canola oil (canola because it is a big GM crop). Choose your healthy cooking oils from the list below. Select them according to the smoke point for the recipe you are preparing. You do not want to overheat your oil or it will oxidize, meaning that you are creating free radicals that will contribute to inflammation in your body. Smoke point means the temperature at which the oil begins to smoke and oxidize. Choose only unrefined, high-quality, organic cold-pressed oils.

- Almond oil is suitable for high-heat cooking with a smoke point of 420 degrees.

- Avocado oil has a medium smoke point of 375 to 400 degrees.

- Virgin organic coconut oil has been used as a traditional remedy for many ailments and is considered to have anti-inflammatory properties. It received quite negative press for several decades, which was completely unfounded and based on marketing schemes by the seed and vegetable oil industry. Only use virgin organic coconut oil because it is processed in a manner that preserves its healthy qualities. It is good for mid-temperature cooking with a smoke point of 350 degrees.

- Extra-virgin olive oil. There is a special compound known as oleocanthal present in olive oil that helps in preventing the production of pro-inflammatory COX-1 and COX-2 enzymes. So when olive oil is used for food preparation, it helps in reducing pain and inflammation. Olive oil is good for medium temperature cooking and has a smoke point around 375 degrees. Oxidation of substances found in extra-virgin olive oil, as well as acrylamide formation, can occur at higher temperatures.

- Ghee (clarified butter, which is butter oil) has a high smoke point of 485 degrees.

- Grape seed oil is suitable for high-heat cooking as well with a smoke point of 420 degrees.

BUYER BEWARE

It used to be that substitution with soybean and sunflower seed oil was the olive oil industry fraud. But one of the big problems now is what they call deodorized oil: oil that has been made out of inedible olives, olives that have been swept up off the ground with what look like street sweepers. You go to agricultural fairs in southern Spain and see a huge range of these different olive pickers—except that they're picking up olives that have been sitting on the ground for a long time.

Then they give them a very light, delicate refining process that doesn't leave very many chemical footprints, so it's very difficult for enforcers to pick it up with standard quality tests. They sell that mixed with real extra-virgin olive oil to give it flavor as extra-virgin. That's because there are chemical requirements for oil to be extra-virgin, but there are also taste requirements; it has to have some fruitiness, and it can't have any defects. This deodorized oil, at least in the first few weeks, is defect free. But it rapidly deteriorates and becomes rancid.[12]

Five tips for recognizing REAL extra-virgin olive oil:

- Be suspicious of any extra-virgin olive oil that costs less than ten dollars a liter.
- Look for a seal from the International Olive Oil Council (IOC).
- Look for a harvesting date on the label.
- Anything labeled light, pure, or a blend isn't virgin quality.[13] Dr. Weston Price group recommends Bariani Extra Virgin Olive Oil.

- Red palm oil has been shown to possess potent antioxidant, anticancer, and cholesterol-lowering activities. It is rich in tocotrienol (a unique form of vitamin E) and has potent anti-inflammatory activity through the inhibition of iNOS and COX-2 production, as well as NF-kappaB expression. It is good for high-heat cooking with a smoke point of 455 degrees.

- Rice bran oil has a smoke point of 490 degrees and is often used for high temperatures such as wok stir-fry.

- Walnut oil, which is anti-inflammatory with its omega-3s, has a low smoke point of 320 degrees.

Additional Guidelines

- Use only healthy sweeteners: stevia (Sweet Leaf Vanilla Creme is very good), coconut sugar and nectar, xylitol made from organic birch bark (but not what is the by-product of the wood pulp industry, which is the majority), and small amounts of raw honey or pure maple syrup.

- Limit acid-forming foods. About 25 percent of your diet should be acid-forming foods (75 percent should be alkaline): 1) whole grains: brown rice, quinoa, millet, spelt, amaranth, and kamut; 2) animal protein: fish, chicken, turkey, and red meat; 3) legumes: beans, lentils, split peas.

- Eat only clean meat and poultry. Not all muscle meat is created equal. In addition to being higher in omega-3 fats and CLA, meat from grass-fed animals is also higher in vitamin E. In fact, studies show the meat from pastured cattle is four times higher in vitamin E than meat from feedlot cattle and, interestingly, almost twice as high as the meat from feedlot cattle given vitamin E supplements. Free-range pastured poultry shows similar benefits.

- Fishing for health. Choose only wild-caught fish. Your choices are limited to wild-caught trout and wild-caught Alaskan salmon, which is regularly tested and found to have no significant level of Fukushima radiation. Avoid farm-raised fish. They are given antibiotics and hormones and are fed very toxic food that can include flame retardants.

- Water. Drink at least sixty-four ounces of purified water to flush out toxins and aid cellular metabolism.

Healing Green Mung Bean Soup

Mung beans provide anti-inflammatory benefits by inhibiting the release of the protein (HMGB1), which regulates inflammatory response. In Ayurveda medicine, mung bean soup is known to help balance the body. Its spices and penetrating herbs are the driving force to help rid the body of toxins and mucus that lodges there over time due to poor diet, lack of exercise, and an unhealthy lifestyle. This soup helps to break down mucus and flush it out of the body.

Preparation time: 45 minutes

1 cup whole green mung beans
2 cups purified water plus ½ tsp sea salt (to cook beans)
1 Tbsp. coconut oil, extra-virgin olive oil, or ghee
½ tsp. mustard seeds
¼ tsp. hing (Eastern spice); optional
1 bay leaf
½ tsp. turmeric
½ tsp. cumin
1–2 tsp. coriander powder
2 cups purified water, for the soup
2 tsp. ginger, finely chopped
1 tsp. garlic, finely chopped
Freshly ground black pepper, to taste
1 tsp. sea salt
2 tsp. fresh lemon juice

Soak the mung beans overnight in purified water. Drain the beans, wash them 2 times, and cook in a pressure cooker or soup pot with the 2 cups water until tender. It takes around 25 minutes if you use a pressure cooker. (The beans have to be tender.) If you use a regular pot, it will take 40 to 45 minutes for the beans to be fully cooked.

Heat the oil or ghee in a large deep soup pot and add mustard seeds. When the mustard seeds pop, add hing, if using, and bay leaf, turmeric, cumin, coriander, ginger, garlic, and a pinch of black pepper. Mix well, sauté, and do not allow to burn.

Place the cooked beans, water, and salt in the soup pot with the herbs and spices. Bring to a boil then simmer for about 15 minutes. Add lemon, remove the bay leaf, and enjoy!

(Adapted from Dr. Oz: http://www.doctoroz.com/recipe/green-mung-bean -soup.)

Why You Should Choose Organic

The popularity of organic foods has increased dramatically in recent years and continues to grow in popularity. Sales of organics reach into the billions of dollars each year and continue to increase annually. There is an ever-growing number of people who want to avoid the billion pounds or more of pesticides and herbicides sprayed onto or added to our crops yearly. That's for good reason! It's estimated that only about 2 percent of this amount actually fights insects and weeds, while the rest is absorbed into the plants and earth and diffused into our air, soil, and water.

When you buy your produce from certified organic farmers, or from local farmers that sell un-sprayed produce but are working without certification, you won't get synthetic fertilizers, sewage sludge, genetically modified organisms, or ionizing radiation. Buying your vegetables from a local source is also the best way to insure freshness. Keep in mind that the fresher the vegetables, the more biophotons (light rays of energy) you'll be receiving. Many local farmers will deliver a box of organic vegetables each week to your home for a reasonable price.

According to results from a $25 million study of organic food, the largest of its kind to date, organic produce completely outshines conventional fare in nutritional content. A four-year European-Union-funded study in 2007 found that organic fruits and vegetables contain up to 40 percent more antioxidants. They have higher levels of beneficial minerals like iron and zinc. Milk from organic herds contained up to 90 percent more antioxidants. The researchers obtained their results after growing fruits and vegetables and raising cattle on adjacent organic and non-organic sites attached to Newcastle University. According to Professor Carlos Leifert, coordinator of the project, eating organic foods can even help to increase the nutrient intake of people who don't eat the recommended number of servings of fruits and vegetables a day.[14]

AVOID THE "DIRTY DOZEN"

If you can't afford to buy all organic produce, you could still avoid the worst pesticide-sprayed foods by using only organically grown produce on the top dozen list. The nonprofit research organization Environmental Working Group (EWG) reports periodically on health risks posed by pesticides in produce. The group says you can cut your pesticide exposure by almost 90 percent simply by avoiding the twelve conventionally grown fruits and vegetables that have been found to be the most contaminated. It has been found that eating the twelve most contaminated fruits and vegetables will expose a person, on average, to about fourteen pesticides per day. Eating the twelve least contaminated conventionally grown fruits and vegetables will expose a person to less than two pesticides per day. Here's the current dirty dozen twelve plus two:

1. Apples
2. Sweet bell peppers
3. Celery
4. Cherry tomatoes
5. Cucumber
6. Grapes
7. Kale/collard greens
8. Nectarines (imported)
9. Peaches
10. Hot peppers
11. Potatoes
12. Spinach
13. Strawberries
14. Summer squash

The list changes each year. To get current ratings, go to www.ewg.org.

Nutrient Recommendations

Antioxidants are powerful free-radical quenchers. Free radicals, produced as part of the inflammatory process, are unstable molecules that damage cells. Damaged cells then become sources of even more free radicals, and a chain reaction is set in motion. Antioxidant nutrients bind to free radicals, preventing them from injuring healthy tissue and thereby reducing the inflammation process. The following antioxidants are quite helpful in keeping inflammation in check:

- Copper has been shown to decrease inflammation in laboratory animals. Best sources of copper include oysters, Brazil nuts, almonds, split peas, buckwheat, ginger root, turnips, parsley, garlic, carrots, spinach, cabbage, lettuce, and cucumbers. You should not need to take additional copper supplementation, except for what comes in a multivitamin/mineral capsule.

- Quercetin is found in fruits and vegetables. It may be as helpful as over-the-counter medications in inhibiting histamine release and stabilizing mast cells, but without side effects such as drowsiness. By inhibiting histamine release at the outset, quercetin stands in direct contrast to many medications that attempt to nullify the effects of histamine after an allergic reaction has already taken place. When combined with the herb nettle, quercetin is helpful to prevent or reduce sneezing, itching, and inflammation of the nasal passages. It also helps prevent vitamin C depletion. For supplemental dose to help reduce inflammation, you could take 500 mg twice a day and up 2,000 mg daily.

- Selenium is a powerful antioxidant. Best sources of selenium include chard, turnips, garlic, radishes, carrots, cabbage, apple cider vinegar, and Brazil nuts (one of the best sources). Four Brazil nuts gives you almost 400 mcg of selenium. For supplemental dose, you could take up to 400 mcg.

- Vitamin A and beta-carotene are potent antioxidants. Beta-carotene is converted to vitamin A in the body as needed. Best sources of carotenes in general include carrots, kale, parsley, spinach, chard, beet greens, watercress, broccoli, and romaine lettuce; cod liver oil is among the best. You do not need to take vitamin A supplements if you take cod liver oil or eat a diet rich in vegetables and fruit.

- Vitamin C and bioflavonoids both inhibit the release of histamine, a substance that is released in response to infections and allergies. In addition, vitamin C stabilizes cell membranes, and bioflavonoids enhance the action of vitamin C. Best sources of vitamin C include kale, parsley, broccoli, brussels sprouts, watercress, cauliflower, cabbage, spinach, lemons, limes, turnips, and asparagus. Best sources of bioflavonoids include bell peppers, berries (blueberry, blackberry, and cranberry), lemons, limes, broccoli, cabbage, parsley, and tomatoes. Recommended supplement dosage of vitamin C is about 2,000 mg per day, but may vary depending on age, health (are you fighting a bug?) and how many vitamin C–rich foods you eat.

- Vitamin E is considered an anti-inflammatory antioxidant. Best sources of vitamin E include almonds, olive oil, spinach, watercress, asparagus, carrots, and tomatoes. Recommended supplement dosage is 400 IUs daily.

- Zinc promotes anti-inflammatory activity. Best sources of zinc include oysters, ginger root, beef, lamb, chicken, turnips, parsley, garlic, carrots, grapes, spinach, cabbage, lettuce, and cucumbers. Recommended supplement dosage is no more than 100 mg. I would not recommend taking extra zinc, other than what is in your multivitamin/ mineral capsule, other than when you have a cold, since long-term use for ten years or more increases the risk of prostate cancer.

Herb and Spice Recommendations

- Ashwaganda is an adaptogenic herb that has antioxidant activity and has also demonstrated anti-inflammatory activity. The recommended dosages is 500 mg daily.

- Boswellia (frankincense), when taken at a dose of 300 mg, three times daily, acts as a powerful anti-inflammatory supplement.

- Burdock is a wonderful digestive herb that supports liver function and detoxification, reduces liver inflammation, heals liver cells in fatty liver disease, and stimulates stomach acid production. Burdock root is a mild-tasting, slow-acting, nourishing medicine. Here's how you can get more burdock root into your diet: cut up sweet potatoes, carrots, beets, kohlrabi, and burdock into bite-sized pieces and put them on a cookie sheet. Toss them in olive oil or coconut oil and sprinkle with garlic salt and a combination of spices such as Spike. Bake at 375 degrees for about 45 minutes. You can also stir-fry with broccoli and onions for a side dish. Or put some chopped burdock in chili or beef or lamb stew.[15] You can also juice it up in your favorite juice recipes.

- Curcumin, a constituent of turmeric, has anti-inflammatory effects. Traditionally it has been used on wounds, sprains, and inflamed joints to decrease inflammation. It is as effective as some prescription drugs in relieving the swelling and stiffness associated with arthritis. Curcumin is available in supplement form. You can also cook with turmeric (which contains curcumin), add it to spicy tea with a bit of ghee, and combine it in a smoothie.

- Dandelion enhances bile flow. It also reduces and prevents inflammation in the liver and gallbladder. You can make dandelion tea by pouring one cup of boiling water over one to two teaspoons of dried dandelion leaves, sauté or steam the leaves, or add them to an omelet or a smoothie. They have a bitter flavor, so you may need to experiment with what works for you. But don't leave them out of your diet; they have many health benefits.

- Devil's claw is similar in its anti-inflammatory effects to cortisone. It also helps relieve pain.

- Garlic. There is evidence that some inflammatory aspects of obesity may be altered by sulfur-containing compounds in garlic.

- Ginger is a powerful anti-inflammatory. Studies identified ginger as an herbal medicinal product that shares pharmacological properties with non-steroidal anti-inflammatory drugs. Ginger suppresses prostaglandin synthesis through inhibition of cyclooxygenase-1 and cyclooxygenase. It can also protect the stomach from the effects of nonsteriodal anti-inflammatory drugs (NSAIDs). Fresh ginger tastes great in almost any juice or smoothie recipe.

Chai Tea

2 tsp. ground ginger
2 tsp. ground cinnamon
1 tsp. ground cloves
1 tsp. ground cardamom
1 tsp. nutmeg
1 tsp. allspice
¼ tsp. white pepper

Mix all ingredients well and keep in a covered container. Mix ½ to 1 teaspoon of the spice mix with 8 ounces hot water. Add 1 teaspoon ghee and stir. This is a very warming tea for autumn and winter.

- Hibiscus. When it comes to antioxidant content, hibiscus has more antioxidant power than green tea. Hibiscus helps lower high blood pressure, lowers uric acid levels in gout sufferers, and improves cholesterol and triglyceride levels in prediabetics and diabetics. You can sip iced hibiscus tea throughout the day. It also acts as a diuretic.

Hibiscus Power Iced Tea

Chopped hibiscus flowers (order from Amazon) or 5 hibiscus herbal tea bags[*]
12 mint leaves (optional)
Juice of 1 lime (optional)
2 quarts purified water

Steep hibiscus tea or flowers in water. I put it all in the refrigerator. In about an hour you have iced tea.

    *I recommend Hibiscus tea or "Back on Tract"—hibiscus and cranberry—both by Traditional Medicinals (visit their website at www.traditionalmedicinals.com).

- Licorice inhibits phospholipase A, an enzyme that, like platelet-activating factor, starts inflammatory reactions. Use whole licorice extract for inflammatory disorders. Do not use licorice candy. Use DGL (have no glycyrrhizin) if you have high blood pressure, kidney or liver disease, diabetes or heart disease, and do not use for more than six weeks. Use licorice if you have low adrenals. I like licorice tea by Traditional Medicinals.

- Magnolia extract. Magnolia bark contains two anti-inflammatory substances, magnolol and honokiol, which reportedly inhibit the activation of NF-KB, a key mediator in both inflammatory and aging processes. The recommended dose is 200 mg daily.

- Parsley contains flavonoids—especially luteolin—that have been shown to combine with highly reactive oxygen-containing molecules (oxygen radicals) and help prevent oxygen-based damage to cells. This means reduction in inflammation.

- Peppermint's essential oil acts as a decongestant, and certain substances in peppermint contain anti-inflammatory and mild antibacterial constituents.

- Rhodiola is considered an adaptogenic herb, meaning that it acts in nonspecific ways to increase resistance to stress without disturbing normal biological functions. Evidence suggests that it acts as an antioxidant and enhances immune system function. Clinical research has shown Rhodiola to enhance cognition, improve memory and learning, greatly reduce stress and fatigue, stimulate the immune system, increase metabolism, aid thyroid function, protect the cardiovascular system, boost fertility and sexual function, and improve mood. It brews a red pink tea that smells and tastes reminiscent of rose petals. Use one to three teaspoons per cup, more for a real cerebral workout. Steep for ten to fifteen minutes; if steeped longer the tea becomes strongly astringent. Mixing it with Rooibos tea is quite delicious and helps to balance the astringency. (Roobios tea helps to naturally reduce high cortisol levels.) Do not drink Rhodiola late in the day as it can keep you awake.[16]

- White willow bark. In combination with the herb's powerful anti-inflammatory plant compounds (flavonoids), salicin is thought to be responsible for the pain-relieving and anti-inflammatory effects of the herb. In the 1800s salicin was used to develop aspirin. White willow appears to bring pain relief more slowly than aspirin, but its effects may last longer.

Other Supplements That Help

- Amylase is a digestive enzyme that breaks down complex carbohydrates into simple sugars. It's also present in saliva. So while we chew our food, it goes to work on carbs. That's why it's recommended that you chew each mouthful of food about thirty times.

- The pancreas makes amylase. And amylase is plentiful in seeds that contain starch. (You can juice most seeds of fruits and vegetables.) Its therapeutic use is in the regulation of histamine, which is produced in response to recognized invaders to the body. Histamine is a responder in allergic reactions such as hay fever and is what causes hives; itchy, watery eyes; sneezing; and runny noses. Amylase breaks down the histamine produced by the body in response to allergens such as pollen or dust mites. Some health professionals believe it may help the body identify the allergen as not being harmful so it doesn't produce the histamine in the first place. This is one reason that people on a high raw-plant diet often experience improvement in their allergies.

- For the most effective approach to increasing enzymes such as amylase, you may want to take an enzyme supplement. I especially like an enzyme formula that is taken between meals. It cleans up any undigested particles of food floating around the system and greatly improves digestion. A popular side benefit is that your hair gets thicker and your nails grow stronger!

- Evening primrose oil is a fatty acid that is a good source of gamma-linolenic acid (GLA), which can help maintain healthy joints by modifying inflammation.

- Probiotics: Toxicity in your gut can flow throughout your body and into your brain, where it can cause symptoms of autism, ADHD, dyslexia, dyspraxia, depression, schizophrenia, and other mental disorders. Reducing gut inflammation is imperative. Hippocrates said all disease begins in the gut. The largest part of your immune system is in your gut. The gastrointestinal tract has a vital role in your health, including digestion, nutrient absorption, defense against invading pathogens, hormone metabolism, detoxification, and elimination and production of energy. Natasha Campbell-McBride, MD, developed the GAPS Diet in her efforts to effectively heal gut-related disorders. She emphasized the importance of detoxifying the intestinal tract, healing the gut through nutrient-dense foods, and sealing or protecting the gut by establishing healthy levels of beneficial bacteria, using traditional fermented foods and beverages. Heal your gut and you take a big step toward putting out the flame of inflammation in your body. Take only human strain probiotics.

- Prebiotic is a specialized plant fiber you find in plant foods that beneficially nourishes the good bacteria already in the large bowel. The body does not digest these plant fibers; instead, the fibers act as a fertilizer to promote the growth of many of the good bacteria in the gut. These, in turn, provide many digestive benefits. Adding foods with nondigestible prebiotic content creates positive changes in the profile of gut bacteria. They reduce inflammation, endotoxemia, insulin resistance, appetite, fat mass, glycemia, lipids, liver inflammation, and increase glucose tolerance.

TOP PREBIOTIC FOODS[17]

1. Asparagus (raw), 5 percent
2. Banana (raw), 1 percent
3. Chicory root (raw), 64.6 percent
4. Dandelion greens (raw), 24.3 percent
5. Garlic (raw), 17.5 percent
6. Jerusalem artichoke (raw), 31.5 percent
7. Leeks (raw), 11.7 percent
8. Onion (raw), 8.6 percent
9. Cooked onion, 5 percent
10. Wheat bran (raw), 5 percent

Detoxify Your Body

You can take anti-inflammatory drugs, swallow fish oil daily, faithfully gulp down supplements, and munch on cacao nibs all year long, but if you don't get rid of pro-inflammatory food and toxins that contribute to your inflammation, you'll simply be pouring good things on top of your toxin and food-fueled inflammation.

You need to do a complete body detox. It's imperative to control parasites, fungus, yeasts, bacteria, and viruses. These pathogens can be hidden sources of inflammation. It's advantageous to periodically do a *Candida albicans* cleanse and a parasite cleanse. Detoxing your body is an excellent ally in eliminating inflammation. See my book *Juicing, Fasting, and Detoxing for Life* for complete detox programs.

Eat, Drink, and Be Well

Now that you know about the foods you want to include in your diet and the foods you want to avoid, it's time to put it all into practice with the recipes in the pages that follow. You are in for a real treat with twenty-eight days of beautiful, delicious, and nurturing foods. My prayer is that at the end of your delicious journey, you'll feel renewed, filled with joy, and healthy. Here's to eating well *and* living well.

Chapter 4

TWENTY-EIGHT DAYS TO VIBRANT HEALTH RECIPES AND MEAL PLAN

The doctor of the future will give no medication, but will interest his patients in the care of the human frame, diet, and in the cause and prevention of disease.[1]

—THOMAS EDISON

O YOU KNOW what's killing most of us in America? Breakfast, lunch, and dinner. That's right! It's what we're eating every day that's causing so much illness and disease in our fast-food, eat-on-the-run society. But this is changing for you. You're leaning how to make the wisest choices possible while also enjoying what you eat. Half the battle is planning ahead and having recipes you enjoy

Your twenty-eight-day menu plan in this chapter not only will help you plan ahead with delicious recipes, but also it will help you reduce inflammation and promote vibrant health. You can jump right in and start your program as soon as you wish. You don't have to do anything special to get started. Your anti-inflammation diet will help you gently detox your body. We encourage you to follow each week's menu plan as much as possible. We have prepared a shopping list to help you collect everything you need for the week. Each week you can make a copy of the shopping list. It's complete with boxes to check off the items as you gather them on Saturday, Sunday, or whenever you do your week's shopping. If you don't want to make all the recipes, there's also a shopping list below each recipe. This makes it easy for you to tailor the plan to your needs.

We also recommend that you shop for local produce whenever possible. Late spring, summer, and fall you'll find an abundance of local and often organic produce at farmer's markets. This is the freshest, healthiest choice you can make. It's life-giving for your soul and body. You're interacting with local farmers who grew the food and display it with pride. This also helps you eat with the seasons—another excellent way to promote good health. In addition to farmer's markets, search out local stores that carry organic produce and healthy ingredients like organic herbs and spices, coconut nectar, and sea salt.

Setting Up for Success in the Kitchen

From Chef Abby

There are several ways to save time while prepping multiple recipes. First, look through the week's recipes and see what items you can prep all at once. For example, destem all your leafy greens, clean them, and have them ready to chop in your fridge lined with towels to keep them dry and fresh. Mince a head of garlic or a piece of ginger, and keep it fresh in your fridge by covering with olive oil. Chop sturdy root vegetables like carrots, sweet potatoes, or parsnips, and cover in water in your fridge so you are ready to cook them midweek. As Cherie will also mention, it's a great idea to pick one day a week to get some bulk prep cooking done so you are priming yourself for success! Once you start chopping and cleaning produce, you will find you save time by doing a lot at once.

The same goes for shopping. Take your weekly list, and plan one (or two) bulk shopping trips. Clean all your produce when you return so you are one step closer to cooking when the time is right. These are life skills that will benefit your health and relationship with cooking long after you complete this twenty-eight day menu plan.

A NOTE ABOUT CERTAIN RECIPE INGREDIENTS

Salt

Sea salt is our preferred salt of choice. It is less processed than regular table salt and often contains trace minerals and elements that are beneficial to overall health. My personal recommendation is to use gray sea salt, Celtic sea salt, true sea salt, or pink salt. I personally use a brand from Utah called Real Salt. You may need to purchase a salt mill if you choose to use a coarse version of any of these salts. But there are fine varieties as well. We do not recommend that you use Morton's sea salt because there is added iodine, and it is heavily processed.

Pepper

I also recommend that you purchase whole black peppercorns and grind (or crack) them fresh for each recipe using a pepper mill. Fresh pepper is detoxifying. The outer layer of the peppercorn stimulates the breakdown of fat cells. Pepper stimulates HLC (hydrochloric acid), which helps with overall digestion.

Olive oil

There are differences between the various types of olive oil. I suggest that you find a quality extra-virgin olive oil for salad dressings, and use regular olive oil for cooking.

Lastly, consider the power of a team. Grab your best friend or spouse, your sister or mom, and have them participate in the twenty-eight-day program with you. Set aside a few days a month to cook with them, prepping dishes together or sharing in the cooking. You will be more accountable to complete the full program, and also you may find yourself enjoying these recipes for years to come, as positive associations with friends and family around the table develop through your commitment to the plan. The buddy system always works.

Prepping for a Juice and Smoothie Takeover!

From Cherie

You may want to choose Saturday or Sunday as a juice and smoothie prep day. There are things you can do ahead of time to make it easier to eat well during the week. For example, many people find it hard to juice each day, but it becomes doable when they make all the juices on the weekend and freeze them in individual containers. Leave some room at the top for expansion, or your jars will break. There are different juice or smoothie recipes for each day of the week. This is to give you a variety of options. You don't have to make a different juice or smoothie each day, however. You can make your favorites and keep it simple.

Photo by Sika Stanton

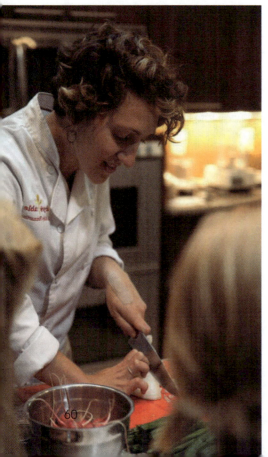

Planning Ahead With Cherie and Abby

When planning your shopping, you may also want to double or even triple amounts if you have a large family or you're preparing a dish for a potluck or extended family get-together. If you're cooking for just yourself, you may want to cut amounts in half. Or you may want to make the full amount and freeze a portion so you'll have meals ready for busy days. We've designed some recipes for that option already with extra food you can use the next day in a recipe. Other days there is extra food you can freeze for future meals. When changing the way you eat, it's important to plan ahead so that you aren't stuck at busy times with nothing to eat and no time to make something. That's when most of us get into trouble. We head for fast food in one form or another. Also, we want you to have a break from time to time and not have to spend much time in the kitchen. If you can make a quick salad and pull a frozen soup or other dish out of the freezer, you've got an easy meal. Start thinking about how you'll make that happen on a regular basis.

The reasoning for the menu plan was to give you guidelines—to show you what an anti-inflammatory diet should look like along with giving you recipes to enjoy. Never feel that you can't take advantage of the program because there is a food or recipe you don't like or can't eat. For example, if you are allergic to eggs, use an egg replacer or make a different recipe. If you don't like one item in a recipe or can't find it, substitute something else. We've both heard from many people who give up because there's one food in a recipe or menu plan they can't eat or don't like. This is the time to get creative. If you can't figure out what to substitute for an item, try doing a search online for substitutes. If the recipe sounds unappealing, search for one that does appear appetizing and stays within the anti-inflammation guidelines. Make this a fun cooking and food prep adventure. You'll be surprised at how innovative you can be.

What's for breakfast? We have a variety of recipes interspersed through the menu plan. You may want only a glass of juice or a smoothie for breakfast. But you may also need some additional food or extra protein to start your day. Look for recipes that work for you. We also have some fun breakfast ideas for weekends like gluten-free pancakes and sweet potato hash. For healthy snacks and desserts, see the sections at the end of Week Four. We want to make sure that you have plenty of snack and dessert ideas that won't cause inflammation in your body.

We're very excited to share our recipes with you not only because we think you'll enjoy them, but also because we know they are health promoting.

Enjoy!

—CHERIE AND CHEF ABBY

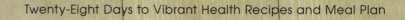
Time-Saving Kitchen Tips From Chef Abby

Chop while you are at it.

When I take the time to clean and chop any vegetable, I always prep more than I need. I save time by being in the chopping "zone" and only needing to clean my countertop and cutting board once for a lot of produce. While you're honing your knife skills, you may as well get right to it.

- Chop extra garlic and keep it fresh for the week by covering it with olive oil and placing in the fridge.

- Chop extra root veggies (carrots, sweet potatoes, rutabaga, pumpkin) and keep covered in water in a glass bowl in the fridge so you are ready to pull them out, boil, and roast them anytime.

- Destem your leafy greens.

- Clean your spinach and lettuces and keep dry with towels in between the layers.

These steps make it easy to whip together a weeknight meal in no time at all.

Designate your bulk day.

One day a week (typically Monday for me) I do some bulk cooking. This is not a new idea, but it's a great one that yields some staples ready to work with for the week. Here are some personal staples:

- Chicken stock (using a whole roasted chicken we have eaten that weekend)

- A batch of quinoa or brown rice

- Roasted or blanched veggies (many kinds, keep it different weekly)

- A jar of salad dressing

- A soup or stew (often using the stock and veggies I just made, or the last of the veggies that need to be utilized before I make a weekly trip to the store)

If you have the time, make a sturdy salad (like a hand-cured kale salad) that can also serve as an easy side to a midweek meal. Once you start, you'll find that bulk cooking doesn't take you as long as you think, since once you get going, you might as well make more.

Finish up, stand in awe of your full fridge, and applaud yourself for the time you will save all week long for the efforts of this day.

Use your halves right away.

I admit it, I also cut halves of veggies and leave them in my fridge thinking they will be used within a few days. Sometimes this just doesn't happen, and that half a sweet potato or onion or bunch of mustard greens you thought you would use is now past its prime. The solution: utilize it right away.

Example:

- If you are using half a pumpkin and half an onion to make a soup, throw the other half (without even seeding it or chopping it further) in the oven on 325, facedown, to roast with some olive oil and the chopped onion around it. Voilà! Once baked, remove the seeds and you have another side dish ready for a meal, and you didn't use any extra prep time to make it.

Cook often so you shop for the right things.

This tip comes from my awesome husband, Eric, who pointed out that

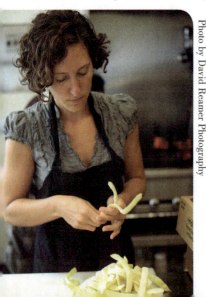

Photo by David Reamer Photography

when you are cooking on a regular cycle as we do, you know exactly what you need when you make the trip to the store. You know that you've used up your last bit of kale, and that nothing is going to waste in your fridge since you've already taken the precious time to make a soup for the week. This is a very insightful addition to this list, since it means that you are going to save money by not (unintentionally) withering good produce simply due to time.

Week One Shopping List

Cooking wine and vinegar

- ❏ Apple cider vinegar
- ❏ Balsamic vinegar
- ❏ Mirin or rice wine vinegar
- ❏ Red wine vinegar
- ❏ Rice vinegar

Dairy and eggs

- ❏ 1½ dozen eggs

Dried fruit

- ❏ 2½ cup unsweetened dried cranberries
- ❏ Dried currants
- ❏ 4 dried mission figs

Dry herbs and spices

- ❏ Bay leaves
- ❏ Black peppercorns (or ground black pepper)
- ❏ Cayenne pepper
- ❏ Celery salt
- ❏ Cinnamon sticks
- ❏ Coriander seeds
- ❏ Dried basil
- ❏ Dried oregano

- ❏ Fennel seeds
- ❏ Ground cinnamon
- ❏ Ground cloves
- ❏ Ground cumin
- ❏ Ground ginger
- ❏ Ground nutmeg
- ❏ Ground turmeric
- ❏ Mustard powder
- ❏ Paprika
- ❏ White pepper

Dry or canned pantry items

- ❏ Capers
- ❏ Coconut aminos or tamari
- ❏ 2 cans coconut milk (15 oz.)
- ❏ Dijon mustard
- ❏ Gluten-free breadcrumbs (or 1 pack rice crackers)
- ❏ Green curry paste (optional)
- ❏ Raw honey
- ❏ Maple syrup
- ❏ Niçoise olives
- ❏ Protein powder
- ❏ Sea salt

- ❏ Vanilla extract
- ❏ Dry white wine (optional)
- ❏ Nutritional yeast

Fresh herbs and spices

- ❏ 16 fresh bay leaves
- ❏ 1 bunch cilantro
- ❏ 2 bunch curly parsley
- ❏ 3 bunch flat leaf parsley
- ❏ 7 inches ginger
- ❏ ¼ cup fresh herb of choice
- ❏ 1 bunch mint
- ❏ 1 bunch tarragon
- ❏ 2 sprigs fresh thyme

Fish, poultry, meat

- ❏ 1 whole chicken, free-range or organic
- ❏ 1½ lb. chicken breasts, boneless skinless
- ❏ ½ lb. fresh lump crabmeat
- ❏ 2 lb. skinless wild salmon fillet
- ❏ ½ lb. smoked salmon
- ❏ 1½ lb. shrimp (or more boneless skinless chicken breasts)

- ❏ 1½ lb. wild sole filets (petrale or dover)
- ❏ 1½ lb. wild tuna steaks (omit for vegan option)

Flours

- ❏ ½ cup almond meal or rice flour
- ❏ Arrowroot or tapioca flour
- ❏ Gluten-free all-purpose flour

Grains and beans

- ❏ Quinoa
- ❏ 2 cups red lentils
- ❏ 1 cup brown basmati rice
- ❏ 1 cup short-grain brown rice
- ❏ 8 cups rolled oats (gluten free)
- ❏ ½ cup northern white beans

Nuts and seeds

- ❏ 1 cup almonds
- ❏ 1 quart almond milk
- ❏ ½ cup cashews
- ❏ 1 Tbsp. chia seeds
- ❏ ½ cup + 1 Tbsp. flaxseeds

❏ 4 cups hazelnuts, pecans, or almonds

❏ ¼ cup sesame seeds

❏ ¼ cup sunflower seeds

Oils

❏ Coconut oil

❏ Extra-virgin olive oil

❏ Grape seed oil

❏ Unrefined sesame oil

Produce

Fruit

❏ 4 avocados

❏ 3 apples of choice

❏ 3 green apples

❏ 2 bananas

❏ 12 lemons (or 1 quart lemon juice)

❏ 1 lime

❏ 1 orange

❏ 1 pear

❏ 1 pineapple

❏ 1 pint berries

Vegetables

❏ 3 bunches asparagus

❏ 14 cups baby spinach (1¼ lb.)

❏ 6 beets (with tops)

❏ 1 broccoli stem

❏ 5 lb. carrots

❏ 2 cauliflower heads

❏ 2 bunches celery

❏ 1 bunch collard greens

❏ 6 cucumbers

❏ 3 heads fennel

❏ 4 heads garlic

❏ 1 cup green beans (or another 1 bunch asparagus)

❏ 7 bunches kale

❏ 1 kohlrabi with leaves

❏ ½ cup mushrooms (¼ lb.)

❏ 4 cups pea shoots or arugula (¼ lb.)

❏ 1 head radicchio

❏ 2 bunches radishes

❏ 1 head red cabbage

❏ 2 small red onions

❏ 1 large head romaine lettuce

❏ 4 lb. rutabaga

❏ 1 Napa or savoy cabbage

❏ 8 yellow onions

❏ 10 large handfuls salad greens

❏ 2 bunches scallions

❏ 1 medium shallot

❏ 3 cups snap peas (½ lb.)

❏ 1 pint sprouts

❏ 6 cups vegetables: bok choy, carrots, scallions, shiitake mushrooms, broccoli, snap peas, mustard greens

Stocks

❏ 5 quarts chicken or vegetable stock (homemade is best!)

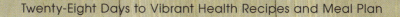
Week One Menu and Recipes

Monday Breakfast

Anti-Inflammatory Cocktail   Serves 2

Fennel: anti-inflammatory, anti-histamine, analgesic, and antioxidant

Apple: inhibits the development of allergies; rich in histamine-lowering quercetin

Cucumber: analgesic (pain killer); antioxidant that prevents the synthesis of the inflammatory compound prostaglandin

Broccoli: anti-carcinogenic, prevents gastric mucosal damage (suggesting potential histamine-lowering action)

Ginger: as effective as an H2 receptor antagonist prescription drug

1 green apple
½ large fennel with fonds
1-inch-piece ginger root
1 large broccoli stem
3 leaves kale
½ cucumber, peeled if not organic

Cut produce to fit your juicer. Start by juicing the apple and finish with the cucumber. Drink as soon as possible.

Shopping List

1 broccoli
1 bunch kale
1 cucumber
1 fennel bulb with fonds
1-inch piece ginger root
1 green apple

Monday Lunch

Hand Cured Summer Chop Vegetables With
Basic Quinoa   Serves 4–6

Hand Cured Summer Chop Vegetables

This recipe keeps well for 4–5 days in the fridge, so make a big batch and enjoy as a crunchy side dish with any meal. Use what vegetables are in season to make this a year round staple.

1 avocado, sliced
1 head (or 4 cups) Napa or savoy cabbage, thinly sliced into bite-size pieces
2 cups snap peas
1 cup green beans, sliced on a bias into thirds
1–2 cups radishes, quartered
2 cloves garlic, minced
2 cups kale, chopped into bite-size pieces
1-inch-piece ginger, minced (optional)
1 tsp. sea salt

Combine all ingredients in a large bowl. With clean hands massage the vegetables as if you are squeezing water out of them. Work the vegetables at least 15 times, then set a plate over top of the bowl. Add weight over top of the plate and set a timer for 10 minutes.

After 10 minutes use the plate to hold the vegetables in the bowl, and tilt to drain the excess liquid into the sink. Work the vegetables another 15 times, and taste. Finish the recipe at this point, or set the plate over top of the bowl 1 more time. Add weight and set timer for 10 minutes.

Repeat the draining process and taste the vegetables. Enjoy many variations on the theme.

Tomatoes are not a great vegetable for this type of salad, as they get mushy with hand working. If you use cucumbers, seed them first.

Variations:
  *Add sesame seeds at the end, or chopped cashews for crunch.
  *Reduce sea salt to ½ teaspoon and add 1 teaspoon umeboshi plum paste.

Basic Quinoa

Combine 1 cup quinoa, 2 cups water, and ¼ teaspoon salt in a medium pot. Bring to a boil over medium-high heat. Once the quinoa boils, cover and reduce heat to low. Simmer for 15 minutes. Turn off heat, keep covered, and steam 5 more minutes. Serves 6.

Shopping List

1 avocado
1 Napa or savoy cabbage
1 head garlic
1-inch-piece ginger
1 cup green beans
1 bunch kale
Quinoa
1 bunch radishes
2 cups snap peas

Check the Pantry

Sea salt

Monday Dinner

Wild Sole Piccata and Roasted Asparagus With a Simple Salad   Serves 4

Wild Sole Piccata

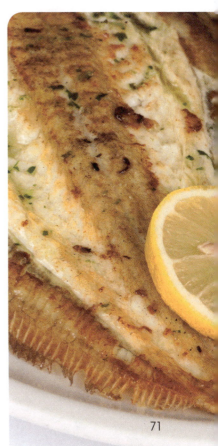

This is a zesty, traditional Italian recipe that is light and refreshing for lunch or dinner. Use almond flour to make it 100 percent grain free.

½ cup almond meal or rice flour
¼ cup nutritional yeast
½ tsp. sea salt, or more to taste
½ tsp. freshly ground black pepper
1½ lb. wild sole filets (petrale or dover)
¼ cup extra-virgin olive oil
¼ cup coconut oil
¼ cup dry white wine (or stock)
¼ cup freshly squeezed lemon juice
¼ cup capers in brine, drained
½ cup fresh parsley, chopped
Additional lemons for garnish and serving
1 large bunch asparagus, tough ends removed
6 handfuls mixed salad greens

Basic Vinaigrette

3 Tbsp. extra-virgin olive oil
2 Tbsp. red wine vinegar (or 1 lemon)
1 clove of garlic
1 tsp. Dijon mustard
½ tsp. raw honey
Sea salt, to taste
Freshly ground black pepper, to taste

In a bowl mix the flour, nutritional yeast, salt, and pepper. If using almond meal, mix the almond flour, yeast, salt, and pepper together. Spread the mixture on a large plate.

Rinse the sole in water and shake off the excess. Dredge 1 filet at a time in the flour mixture, gently pressing the mixture onto the sole. Place on a separate plate while you dredge all the pieces.

Heat a large skillet over medium high heat. Add the olive oil and 2 table-spoons of coconut oil. Once the oil is hot and melted, place 2–3 prepared sole filets in the pan—do not over crowd! Cook for 2–3 minutes or until the first side is well browned. Flip and cook for 2–3 minutes on the other side. Remove cooked sole to a clean serving dish and cover with foil to keep warm. You can also place the plate in a warm oven. Repeat procedure with the remaining pieces.

Add the wine (or stock) and lemon juice to the pan. Scrape the pan to incor-porate all the browned bits left from cooking the fish. Add the capers and cook until the sauce is reduced by about half. It should be the consistency of light syrup. Stir in the remaining 2 tablespoons coconut oil, until melted, and add in parsley. Pour the sauce over the fish, and serve with lemon slices or wedges.

Simple Roasted Asparagus and a Simple Salad

Heat oven to 425. Toss asparagus with olive oil to coat, and sprinkle with salt, pepper, and a touch of balsamic vinegar. Roast for 10 minutes. Toss the basic vin-aigrette with salad greens in a bowl, adding just enough to coat the leaves nicely. Done!

Shopping List	Check the Pantry
½ cup almond meal or rice flour	Black peppercorns
1 large bunch asparagus	Capers in brine
1 clove garlic	Coconut oil
Lemon juice (2 lemons or ¼ cup juice)	Dijon mustard
11 bunches curly parsley	Dry white wine (or stock)
6 handfuls mixed salad greens	Extra-virgin olive oil
½ lb. wild sole filets (petrale or dover)	Nutritional yeast
	Raw honey
	Red wine vinegar (or lemon juice)
	Sea salt

Tuesday Breakfast

Ginger Twist   Serves 1

Ginger has been shown in scientific studies to have anti-inflammatory properties.

1 handful parsley
½ lemon, peeled
4 carrots, scrubbed well, green tops removed, ends trimmed
1-inch-piece fresh ginger root, peeled

Cut produce to fit your juicer's feed tube. Juice ingredients and stir. Pour into a glass and drink as soon as possible.

Shopping List

4 carrots
1-inch-piece ginger root
1 lemon
1 bunch parsley

Tuesday Lunch

Tuna Niçoise Salad With Dijon Vinaigrette   Serves 4

This is a "composed salad" in a traditional sense, so take the time to make each element delicious and arranged beautifully. It's worth the effort!

Dijon Vinaigrette

2 Tbsp. lemon juice
2 Tbsp. Dijon mustard
1 Tbsp. honey
2 Tbsp. apple cider vinegar
1 medium shallot, minced
1 garlic clove, finely minced
¾ cup extra-virgin olive oil
Sea salt
Freshly ground black pepper, to taste

Whisk all ingredients except the oil in a medium bowl. Gradually whisk in the oil. Season to taste with salt and pepper.

Tuna Niçoise Salad

¾ lb. rutabaga, scrubbed and cut into two inch wedges
Sea salt
2 Tbsp. extra-virgin olive oil
1 large head romaine lettuce, leaves washed, rinsed, and torn into bite-sized pieces
1 cup green beans or asparagus, stems removed and halved
Freshly ground black pepper
1½ lb. wild tuna steaks (omit for vegan option)
½ small red onion, sliced very thin
3 hard-boiled eggs, peeled and quartered
¼ cup niçoise olives
1 Tbsp. capers, rinsed

In a large pot, cover rutabaga with 2–3 inches of water. Add 1 tablespoon salt and cook until potatoes are tender, about 8 minutes. Reserve the cooking water. Transfer rutabaga to a medium bowl and toss with a few splashes of olive oil. Set aside.

While the rutabaga is cooking, set the lettuce on serving plates (or in a glass container to pack your lunch).

Bring the reserved water back to a boil and cook green beans (or asparagus) 2 minutes until tender. Drain and submerge in ice cold water for a few minutes. Remove, pat dry, and toss the beans in 1 tablespoon of the vinaigrette, adding salt and pepper to taste. Arrange green beans in a mound at the edge of the lettuce bed.

Heat a large skillet on medium high heat and cook the salmon or tuna steaks 3–4 minutes on each side until cooked medium rare. Remove from pan, and when ready to handle, slice the fish and coat with more of the vinaigrette. Arrange the fish over the lettuce.

Toss the red onion in a bowl and drizzle with a little vinaigrette. Arrange next to the green beans.

Finally slice the hard-boiled eggs and arrange over lettuce and add the olives and capers overtop of the salad.

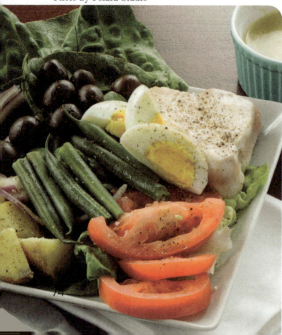

Photo by Polara Studio

Shopping List

¾ lb. rutabaga
1½ lb. wild tuna steaks (omit for
    vegan option)
1 large head romaine lettuce
1 small red onion, sliced very
    thin
3 eggs
1 cup green beans or 1 bunch
    asparagus
1 lemon
1 medium shallot
1 clove garlic

Check the Pantry

Apple cider vinegar
Black peppercorns
Capers
Dijon mustard honey
Extra-virgin olive oil
Niçoise olives
Sea salt

Tuesday Dinner

Basic Asian Stir-Fry With Baked Coriander Brown Rice   Serves 4

Basic Asian Stir-Fry

Make this recipe with a variety of vegetable and protein combinations. This is truly a recipe to play with. Make it once a week for a simple supper. Keep it colorful!

1½ lb. boneless chicken/
    shrimp
5–6 cups thinly sliced
    vegetables, such as
    carrots, bok choy,
    mustard greens, shiitake
    mushrooms, burdock root,
    cooked pumpkin, snap
    peas, scallions, broccoli,
    and broccoli stems
2 Tbsp. coconut oil
1–2 cloves minced garlic
½ inch minced ginger
4 Tbsp. stock (vegetable or
    chicken)

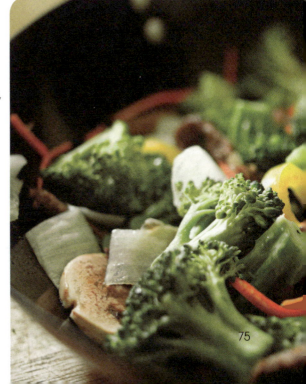

Basic Asian Marinade

1–2 Tbsp. coconut aminos (or tamari)
2 tsp. arrowroot (or tapioca flour)
2 Tbsp. mirin (rice wine vinegar)

If using a protein, cut meat or poultry into 2-inch long pieces less than ½ inch wide. Mix the marinade in a bowl with a whisk to blend. Marinate the chicken or shrimp for 10–20 minutes.

Chop vegetables into bite size pieces (slice on bias). Heat the coconut oil in a large skillet or a wok over very high heat. When the oil begins to ripple stir in the meat or seafood, leaving marinade in the bowl for later use. When meat begins to brown, add the garlic and ginger for 15 seconds, then add the vegetables.

Quickly stir the vegetables and chicken/shrimp until both are done, about 3–5 minutes only. Drain off excess oil from the bottom of the pan and stir in the stock. Simmer for 30 seconds only. Add 1 tablespoon of the marinade into the mixture, stirring for 30 seconds more. Season with coconut aminos or tamari for a saltier flavor.

Optional add-ins: 1 teaspoon sesame oil, 2 teaspoons raw honey, 2 teaspoons lime juice, 1 teaspoon hot chile oil, ¼ cup cashews. Add these ingredients at the end of cooking as you add in the broth or water.

Shopping List

1½ lb. boneless chicken or
   shrimp
½ head garlic
1-inch ginger
Mustard greens
6 cups vegetables: bok choy,
   carrots, scallions, shiitake
   mushrooms, broccoli, snap
   peas

Check the Pantry

Arrowroot or tapioca flour
Coconut aminos or tamari
Coconut oil
Mirin or rice wine vinegar
Vegetable or chicken stock

Baked Coriander Brown Rice   Serves 8

This is a great hands-off way to make aromatic rice using the oven rather than a pot or rice cooker. My favorite version includes a couple cinnamon sticks and coriander seeds! Baking the rice infuses the grain with a nutty aroma. If you soak the rice, reduce the water in this recipe to 4 cups and follow the shorter cooking time listed below.

6 cups water (4 cups for soaked rice)
2 cups brown basmati rice (or short-grain
   brown rice)
2 Tbsp. coriander seeds (or 1 cinnamon stick,
   or seasoning of choice)
¾ tsp. sea salt

Preheat oven to 375 degrees.

Bring the water to a boil in a pot on the stove. Use olive oil to oil a baking dish. Once water boils, add to baking dish, then stir in rice, seasonings, and salt. Cover with foil or a tight fitting lid (foil recommended)

Bake for 50 minutes (basmati rice) or 60–75 minutes for brown rice. If the rice was soaked, bake for 50–60 minutes. Otherwise bake for 75 minutes.

Remove from oven to steam 3–5 minutes. Taste and serve!

Shopping List

2 cups brown basmati rice or
short-grain brown rice

Check the Pantry

Coriander seeds or cinnamon sticks
Sea salt

Wednesday Breakfast

Goin' Green   Serves 1–2

Kale is packed with calcium in a form that is assimilated by the body far better than the calcium in dairy products—and that's a great bonus for your bones!

1–3 kale leaves
1–3 beet leaves
2 stalks celery
1 cucumber, peeled if not organic
3 carrots
1 pear
½ lemon, peeled if not organic

Place some green leaves in your juicer; alternate leaves with celery followed by cucumber, carrot, pear, and lemon. Stir the juice and drink as soon as possible.

Shopping List

1 beet with leaves (use the
beetroot for something else)
1 bunch kale
1 bunch celery
3 carrots
1 cucumber
1 lemon
1 pear

Wednesday Breakfast

Overnight Soaked Muesli With Banana   Serves 4–6

The inspiration for this recipe comes from Jamie Oliver, one of my personal food heroes. This is a great recipe to make with kids, especially since all the prep happens the night before and it's easy and satisfying to finish quickly in the morning.

8 cups organic rolled oats
½ cup flaxseed, whole or ground
2 cups unsweetened raisins, dried cherries, or currants
2 cups chopped nut of choice (toasted)
1 tsp. ground cinnamon
3–4 cups almond or coconut milk, to cover oats
2–3 apples
2 bananas
Raw honey (optional garnish)
Fresh berries (optional garnish)

Put all dry ingredients into a large glass, Tupperware, or gallon bag to combine.

The night before you want to eat your muesli, put your desired portions of the oat mixture into a bowl and cover with almond or coconut milk.

Grate ½ apple per person. Stir in immediately to keep apple from discoloring. Cover and place in the fridge overnight.

In the morning when you're ready to eat it, slice or mash ½ banana per person, stir into the soggy oats and add more almond milk and option raw honey overtop, to taste.

Great served with fresh mixed berries.

Shopping List	Check the Pantry
3–4 cups almond or coconut milk, to cover oats	Cinnamon
	Flaxseed, whole or ground
2–3 apples	Nut of choice
2 bananas	Organic rolled oats
Fresh berries (optional garnish)	Raw honey
	Unsweetened raisins, dried cherries, or currants

Wednesday Lunch

Cream of Carrot Soup With Brown Rice Onigiri With Toasted Nori   Serves 4–6

Cream of Carrot Soup

This is a recipe I adapted from cooking school (the Natural Gourmet Institute of Food and Health in Manhattan). I love the technique of adding cooked grain into the soup to make a creamy finish. Add double ginger if you, like me, love a good kick to your soup!

2 Tbsp. extra-virgin olive oil
1 yellow onion, medium chop
¾ tsp. sea salt
2 lbs. carrots, cut into ½-inch pieces
5 cups of vegetable stock
¼ cup cooked rice or raw cashews, soaked 30 minutes
2-inch-piece of ginger, peeled and chopped
1 Tbsp. lemon juice
Freshly ground black pepper, to taste

Heat a stock pot over medium heat, and add the olive oil. Add the onions and salt, sautéing for 5 minutes. Add the carrots and cover, cooking for another 5 minutes over medium heat. Add the vegetable stock and the cooked rice or cashews to the pot, and bring it to a boil. After the soup starts to boil, reduce the heat and simmer for 25 minutes.

Puree the soup in batches, being careful not to over fill the blender (a hot mess will happen!). Add the fresh chopped ginger into the soup as you puree. Stir in the lemon juice, and season with salt and pepper to taste.

Note: Add more stock if you prefer your soup thinner (add at the end).

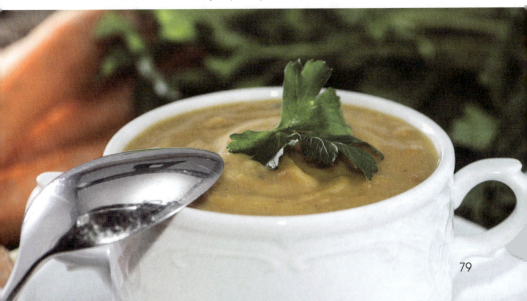

Shopping List

2 lb. carrots
2-inch-piece of ginger
1 lemon (for juice)
2 quarts vegetable stock

Check the Pantry

Black peppercorns
Brown rice or cashews
Extra-virgin olive oil
Sea salt
Yellow onion

Brown Rice Onigiri With Toasted Nori   Serves 6–8

Don't be intimidated by the number of steps! Once you master how to make sticky rice easily, the rest is a cinch. Great for food on the go, onigiri are traditionally served in Japan as an easy lunch or portable meal. Make ahead and serve with many types of meals.

1 cup short-grain brown rice, soaked 4 hours or overnight
2¼ cup filtered water
½ tsp. sea salt
¼ cup rice vinegar
1 Tbsp. sesame oil
¼ cup sesame seeds (optional)
½ cup raw cashews pieces
2 pieces toasted nori, cut into ½-inch by 4-pieces
¼ cup whole umeboshi plums, pitted (optional)

Rinse the soaked rice 3 times by first draining off the soaking liquid, and filling a pot with rice and plenty of water to cover, rubbing the rice with your hands well so the liquid turns a white starchy color. Rinse the water out by tipping the pot, careful to not lose the rice! Fill the pot again with water and repeat twice more. This step makes the rice nice and sticky in a traditional sense.

Now you are ready to cook the rice: Add 2¼ cups water to the soaked and rinsed rice (be sure no rinse water remains) and add the salt. Bring to a boil, cover, then reduce the heat and simmer for 35 minutes. Turn off the heat and allow the rice to steam for 5 minutes.

Spread the rice out on a baking sheet to cool quickly, enough that you can work it with your hands. Sprinkle the rice evenly with rice vinegar and oil.

Pulse the cashews in a food processor until evenly chopped and sprinkle over the rice. Place the rest of the rice vinegar in a small bowl so you can use it to keep your hands moist for rolling.

Grab a bit of sea salt and rub your hands together. Take about a ⅓ up of the rice mixture, and roll into small rice balls, moistening your hands as needed with the vinegar as you go to prevent sticking. Add more salt when desired. Repeat until rice is finished. Sprinkle top with sesame seeds and wrap the nori across the diameter of the rice ball, placing it seam side down until ready to eat. You can stuff the onigiri with optional ingredients such as pickled umeboshi plums or mix chopped pieces into the rice before rolling. Serve at room temperature or chill and enjoy straight out of the fridge. Delicious!

Shopping List

1 cup short-grain brown rice

Check the Pantry

Raw cashew pieces
Rice vinegar
Sea salt
Sesame seeds (optional)
Unrefined sesame oil

Wednesday Dinner

Nut-Crusted Chicken With Whole Roasted Cauliflower and Scallion Cabbage Slaw   Serves 4

Nut-Crusted Chicken

This recipe satisfies the desire for crispy, crunchy, fried food without all the bad oils and white flour. I live in Oregon, so hazelnuts (filberts) are a favorite nut choice for me. Pecans and almonds are also fabulous in this recipe.

2 cups nut of choice, finely ground
1 tsp. sea salt
¼ tsp. freshly ground black pepper
2 tsp. herbs/spices of choice (onion powder, garlic powder, paprika, oregano, etc.)
4 free-range chicken breasts, boneless, skinless, cut in tender-size strips
2 large eggs, beaten

Pour cup of nut meal into a bowl. Add salt, pepper, and enough seasonings until it tastes good to you. Dip the chicken pieces into a beaten egg. Next, lightly coat in nut/seasoning mixture.

Broil on high for 7 minutes, then flip and broil for another 5 minutes, or until juices run clear and there is no pink in the center.

Shopping List

4 large chicken breasts,
    boneless, skinless
2 eggs
2 cups nuts of choice (hazelnut,
    pecan, or almond)

Check the Pantry

Black peppercorns
Herbs/spices of choice
Sea salt

Whole Roasted Cauliflower   Serves 4

2 whole heads of cauliflower, cut in half
¼ cup grape seed oil
½ tsp. sea salt

Preheat the oven to 350 degrees.

Place the cauliflower halves on a lightly oiled baking sheet. Rub the remaining oil on the cauliflower and sprinkle with sea salt.

Roast in the oven for 1 hour. Serve warm or chill and toss in a salad.

Shopping List	Check the Pantry
2 cauliflower heads	Grape seed oil
	Sea salt

Scallion Cabbage Slaw   Serves 4–6

1 head red cabbage, core removed and sliced thinly
3 carrots, matchstick cut
¼ bunch parsley, mint or cilantro
1 bunch of scallions, thinly sliced
1-inch-piece of ginger or 1 clove of garlic, minced
¼ cup apple cider vinegar or lemon juice
½ tsp. sea salt
1 tsp. extra-virgin olive oil (optional)
Freshly ground black pepper or cayenne pepper, to taste (optional)

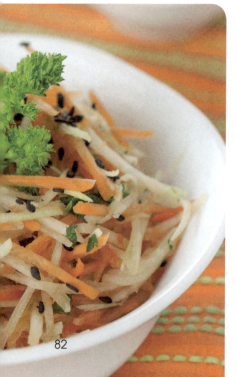

Combine ingredients in a bow. With clean hands massage the salad firmly, squeezing handfuls at a time. Repeat 20 times altogether. Salad should decrease in size and be coated evenly with the dressing.

Taste and adjust the seasonings to taste. Add raw honey to reduce the tartness, add various spices for variety, add more vinegar or salt for a brighter salad. Keep in the fridge for up to 5 days.

Shopping List

3 carrots
1-inch-piece ginger or 1 garlic
   clove
1 bunch mint, cilantro, or
   parsley
1 head red cabbage
1 bunch scallions

Check the Pantry

Apple cider vinegar
Black peppercorns or cayenne
   pepper
Extra-virgin olive oil
Raw honey
Sea salt

Thursday Breakfast

Cherie's Awesome Green Smoothie   Serves 2

Research has identified more than 45 different flavonoids in kale. With kaempferol and quercetin at the top of the list, kale's flavonoids and antioxidants have anti-inflammatory benefits that help us avoid chronic inflammation and oxidative stress.

1 avocado, peeled and seeded and cut in quarters
1 cup baby spinach
2 kale leaves
½ cucumber, peeled and cut in pieces
Juice of 1 lime
1 Tbsp. green powder of choice (optional)
2–3 Tbsp. ground almonds (optional)

Combine all ingredients in a blender and blend well until smooth. Sprinkle ground almonds on top, as desired.

Shopping List

1 avocado
1 bunch kale
1 bunch spinach
1 lime
1 organic cucumber

Check the Pantry

Almonds (if using)

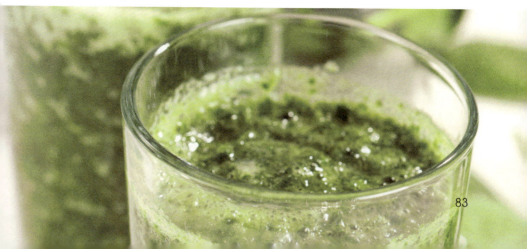

Thursday Lunch

Smoked Salmon Collard Wrap With Honeyed Carrots
Serves 4

Smoked Salmon Collard Wrap

1 large bunch collard greens (8 leaves)
1 avocado, mashed
3 Tbsp. lemon juice, to taste
½ lb. smoked salmon, flaked into pieces
1 cup sprouts
1 cup cucumber, sliced thinly
½ cup tarragon or parsley, chopped
Sea salt, to taste
Freshly ground black pepper, to taste

Assemble the wrap as follows: Destem collard leaf to remove hard central stem so that each collard leaf yields 2 collard wrap pieces.

Lay out the 8 collard leaf pieces in a row and add mashed avocado and a sprinkle of lemon to each piece. Add smoked salmon dividing equally over the avocado.

Add sprouts, cucumber, and tarragon or parsley over the salmon. Roll each piece away from you, carefully placing wrap seam side down, and repeat. Secure with a toothpick until ready to serve.

Shopping List

1 avocado
1 bunch collard greens
1 cucumber
1 bunch parsley or tarragon
½ lb. smoked salmon
1 cup sprouts (alfalfa or your favorite)

Check the Pantry

Black peppercorns
Lemon juice
Sea salt

Honeyed Carrots   Serves 4

1½ lb. carrots, rolling stew cut
½ tsp. sea salt
¼ tsp. freshly ground pepper
½ cup raw honey
2 Tbsp. coconut oil

Wash the carrots then cut: slice on the bias, then roll the carrot away from you, then cut on the bias again. This should form a stew cut carrot. Repeat with remaining carrots.

Place carrots in a skillet and add water to cover halfway up the side of the pan. Cover and steam on high until most of the water evaporates and carrots are nearly steamed through, about 5–7 minutes.

Add remaining ingredients and lower heat to medium low, simmering for 5–10 minutes more until carrots are nicely glazed. Serves 4.

Shopping List

1½ lb. carrots

Check the Pantry

Black peppercorns
Coconut oil
Raw honey
Sea salt

Thursday Dinner

Lemon Lentil Soup With Simple Green Salad and Fig Balsamic Dressing   Serves 6–8

Lemon Lentil Soup

This is one of my most popular soups. It's brightly seasoned with lots of lemon and turmeric, making it an anti-inflammatory favorite. I adapted this recipe from cooking school, where I learned many health supportive recipes. Serve with a dollop of plain coconut yogurt and cilantro pistou (recipe below).

3 Tbsp. coconut oil or extra-virgin olive oil
3 medium onions, finely chopped
3 medium garlic cloves, minced
1–2 carrots, finely chopped
4 stalks celery, finely chopped
¼ heaping tsp. ground cloves
1½ heaping tsp. ground cumin
1–2 Tbsp. turmeric
2 cups red lentils, washed and drained
7 cups water or vegetable stock
2 bay leaves
1-inch lemon zest, cut into thin strips, about 4 pieces
¾ cup lemon juice, or more to taste
2 tsp. sea salt
½ bunch cilantro, coarsely chopped

In a medium saucepan, heat olive oil over medium-high heat and sauté onion, garlic, carrot and celery until soft, 5 minutes. Add ground cloves and cumin; sauté for 1 minute more. Add lentils, water/stock, bay leaves, and lemon zest strips. Bring to a boil, cover, lower heat, and simmer 45 minutes to 1 hour, until lentils are tender but not mushy. Add lemon juice and sea salt. Stir and cook for 3 minutes.

Garnish with chopped cilantro. Alternatively, pulse cilantro with ¼ teaspoon sea salt to create a "pistou" garnish for your soup. Serves 6–8.

Shopping List

- 2 carrots
- ½ bunch celery
- 1 bunch cilantro
- 3 garlic cloves (½ head)
- 4 lemons
- 2 cups red lentils
- 2 quarts vegetable stock
- 3 yellow onions

Check the Pantry

- Bay leaves (fresh)
- Coconut oil or extra-virgin olive oil
- Ground cloves
- Ground cumin
- Ground turmeric

Simple Green Salad With Fig Balsamic Dressing   Serves 4

1 head green leaf lettuce or 4 handfuls baby spinach
½ cup plus 2 Tbsp. extra-virgin olive oil
½ cup balsamic vinegar
4 dried figs, stems removed
½ tsp. sea salt
¼ tsp. freshly ground black pepper
1–2 cloves garlic

Blend all ingredients in a blender or food processor until smooth. Season to taste and toss enough dressing to lightly coat the salad. Serves 4.

Shopping List

- 2 cloves garlic
- 1 head green leaf lettuce or 4 handfuls baby spinach
- 4 dried mission figs

Check the Pantry

- Balsamic vinegar
- Black peppercorns
- Extra-virgin olive oil
- Sea salt

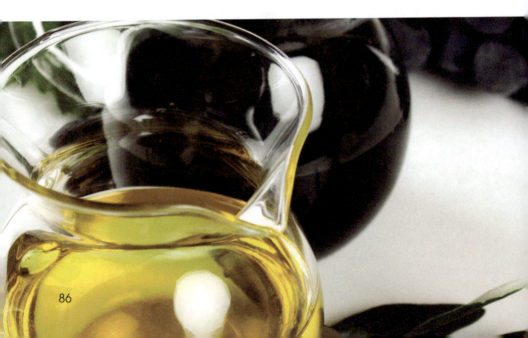

Friday Breakfast

Happy Mood Morning   Serves 1–2

Fennel juice has been used as a traditional tonic to help the body release endorphins, the "feel good" peptides from the brain into the bloodstream. Endorphins help to diminish anxiety and fear and generate a mood of euphoria. 4–5 carrots, well-scrubbed, green tops removed, ends trimmed

3 fennel stalks; include leaves and flowers
½ cucumber
½ apple (green is lower in sugar)
Handful spinach
1-inch-piece ginger root

Cut produce to fit your juicer's feed tube. Juice apple first and follow with other ingredients. Stir and pour into a glass; drink as soon as possible.

Shopping List

4–5 carrots
1 cucumber
1 fennel bulb
1 piece ginger root
1 green apple
1 bunch spinach

Friday Lunch

Basic Raw Kale Salad With Cream of Asparagus Soup
Serves 4–6

Basic Raw Kale Salad

1 cup shredded carrot, or snap peas (when in season)
2 cups radishes, sliced
1 clove garlic, minced
6 cups kale, chopped into bite-size pieces (2 bunches)
1-inch-piece of ginger, minced (optional)
Sea salt, to taste
2 Tbsp. lemon juice
1 Tbsp. extra-virgin olive oil

Combine all ingredients in a large bowl. With clean hands, massage the vegetables as if you are squeezing water out of them. Work the vegetables at least 15 times.

After 10 minutes, work the vegetables another 15 times. Season to taste and enjoy many variations on this theme!

Fun Variations:

*Add sesame seeds and sesame oil at the end, or chopped cashews for crunch.

*Reduce sea salt to ½ teaspoon, and add 1 teaspoon umeboshi plum paste.

*Add golden raisins soaked in apple juice and pumpkin seeds for a kale "granola"!

Shopping List	Check the Pantry
1 clove garlic	Extra-virgin olive oil
1-inch ginger	Sea salt
2 large bunches of kale (green or red or lacinato)	
1 lemon	
1 large bunch radishes	
1 cup snap peas or 3 carrots	

Cream of Asparagus Soup   Serves 6

¼ cup extra-virgin olive oil
2 cloves garlic, chopped
½ cup diced onion
½ Tbsp. green curry paste (optional)
5 cups fresh asparagus, cut into 1-inch pieces (2 bunches)
4 cups rutabaga, one inch dice
4 cups vegetable stock, to cover
¼ bunch parsley, roughly chopped
1½ tsp. sea salt (or more to taste)
Freshly ground black pepper, to taste
1–2 cups coconut milk, or to taste
Fresh water, as needed

Heat the olive oil in a large soup pot set over medium heat and stir in the garlic, onion, and curry paste (this seasons the oil). Add in the cut asparagus and rutabaga. Add *just* enough stock to cover the vegetables—not too much, you can always thin the soup later if you need to.

Add the chopped parsley. Season with sea salt and fresh pepper, to taste. Bring the vegetables to a high simmer. Cover the pot, and reduce the heat to a medium simmer. Cook for 20 minutes or so, until the rutabaga are fork tender.

Remove the pot from the heat. Use an immersion blender to puree the soup. Return the pot to the stove and add in the coconut milk. Stir and heat through gently (don't boil the pureed soup). Taste test and adjust seasonings.

Serve with a sprinkle of fresh minced parsley or a spoonful of plain vegan yogurt or sour cream.

Shopping List

2 bunches asparagus
2 cloves garlic, chopped
1 medium yellow onion
1 bunch parsley
3 lb. rutabaga

Check the Pantry

Black peppercorns
Coconut milk
Extra-virgin olive oil
Green curry paste (optional)
Sea salt
Vegetable stock

Friday Dinner

White Bean Salad With Radicchio and Honeyed Balsamic Dressing With Greek Roasted Beets With Lemon   Serves 4

White Bean Salad With Radicchio

This is a favorite complete meal salad. Heating the salad dressing is a great fall and winter technique to take the raw edge off of sturdy vegetables, and to slightly wilt greens without cooking.

½ lb. dry northern white beans, soaked overnight
2 bay leaves
3 black peppercorns
¼ head fennel (fronds reserved)
2 cloves garlic, minced
½ yellow onion, small diced
½ head radicchio, slice thinly
2 cups pea shoots (use arugula, if unavailable)
1 handful fresh basil
Small handful of pine nuts

Honeyed Balsamic Dressing

¼ cup balsamic vinegar
¼ cup extra-virgin olive oil
1 tsp. dried basil
2 Tbsp. honey
½ tsp. sea salt
Freshly ground black pepper, to taste

Drain and rinse soaked beans. Cook beans al dente: Cover beans with fresh water; add bay leaves, peppercorns, fennel fronds (not chopped fennel). Bring beans to a boil, skim off foam with a spoon. Reduce heat to low, and simmer for 30 minutes.
    Meanwhile, dice up your garlic, onion, and fennel. Set aside. Thinly slice the radicchio, and coarsely chop the pea shoots. Place in a large mixing bowl. Chiffonade basil and reserve in a small bowl (roll basil leaves and very thinly slice to make long ribbons). Whisk the dressing and season to taste.

Once beans are cooked al dente, carefully strain out water and remove the seasonings. Spread beans on a baking sheet to speed up cooling time (5–10 minutes).

Pour dressing into a wide skillet, and bring to a simmer. Add the garlic, onion, and fennel and simmer 3–4 minutes. Add cooled beans to radicchio and pea shoots. Add dressing over top and toss to coat, seasoning with salt and pepper to taste. Add fresh basil, and garnish with pine nuts.

Shopping List	Check the Pantry
1 head fennel	Balsamic vinegar
2 cloves garlic	Basil, dried
1 yellow onion	Bay leaves
2 cups pea shoots or arugula	Black peppercorns
1 head radicchio	Extra-virgin olive oil
½ cup dry northern white beans	Honey
	Sea salt

Greek Roasted Beets With Lemon   Serves 4

A former kitchen volunteer, Annalise, shared with me a recipe she found in a newspaper for "church style" Greek Glazed Potatoes. I adapted it, replacing the average white potato with the gorgeous, healthful beet. The result is this fantastic lemony recipe reminiscent of pickled beets, without sugar added.

3 lb. red beets
½ cup extra-virgin olive oil
½ cup lemon juice
2 Tbsp. Dijon mustard
1½ tsp. sea salt
2 Tbsp. fresh oregano or thyme
1½ tsp. dried oregano
½ tsp. freshly ground black pepper
Water

Quarter the beets lengthwise (cut them into 6–8 pieces if they are large). In a bowl stir together the olive oil, lemon juice, mustard, salt, oregano, and pepper.

Arrange beets cut side up in a large baking pan. Pour the mixture evenly over

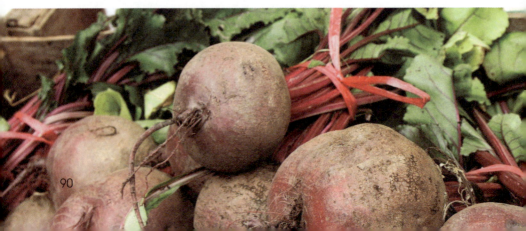

the potatoes. Add enough water to the pan to almost cover the beets (leave about ¼ of the beets uncovered).

Cover with foil and bake on 425 for 1 hour. Uncover and return the beets to oven to continue baking for 30 minutes to glaze, stirring once. Serve hot or cold with extra fresh herbs added, as desired.

Shopping List	Check the Pantry
6 beets	Black peppercorns
4 lemons	Dijon mustard
2–3 sprigs oregano or thyme	Dried oregano
	Extra-virgin olive oil
	Sea salt

Saturday Breakfast

Chia Mia   Serves 2

This combination of omega-3 fatty acids, high-lignan content, and mucilage gums in flaxseeds makes this an excellent anti-inflammatory food.

10 raw almonds
1 Tbsp. raw sunflower seeds
1 Tbsp. chia seeds
1 Tbsp. sesame seeds
1 Tbsp. flaxseeds
1 pineapple or 1 cup unsweetened juice
1 cup chopped parsley
½ cup almond milk
½ tsp. pure vanilla extract
1 Tbsp. protein powder (optional)
6 ice cubes

Place the nuts, seeds, and pineapple juice in a bowl. Cover and soak overnight. Place the nut and seed mixture with the juice in a blender and add the parsley, milk, vanilla, protein powder (if using), and ice cubes. Blend on high speed until smooth. This drink will be a bit chewy because of the nuts and seeds.

Note: To kill molds, add ½ tsp. ascorbic acid to juice, then add nuts and soak overnight.

Shopping List

10 almonds
Unsweetened almond milk
1 package chia seeds or 1 Tbsp.
   chia seeds
1 package flaxseeds, golden or
   brown, or 1 Tbsp. flaxseeds
1 bunch parsley
1 pineapple or 1 cup
   unsweetened juice
1 package sesame seeds or 1
   Tbsp. sesame seeds
1 package of raw sunflower
   seeds or 1 Tbsp. sunflower
   seeds

Check the Pantry

Pure vanilla extract
Protein powder (optional)

Saturday Lunch

Poached Wild Salmon Over Spinach Salad   Serves 6

Poaching Liquid

3 cups water
3 sprigs fresh parsley
1 Tbsp. fennel seeds
2 bay leaves (fresh or dried)
1 cup dry white wine (Pinot Grigio or Sauvignon Blanc)
4 black peppercorns
¾ tsp. sea salt
2 lb. skinless wild salmon fillet
½ cup balsamic vinegar
½ cup extra-virgin olive oil
Freshly ground black pepper, to taste
8 cups spinach greens
1 yellow beet, matchstick cut
½ cup dried currants
¼ cup sunflower seeds

Bring the water to a boil in a pot or deep skillet. Add parsley, fennel, and bay leaves. Remove from the heat and cover to steep for 10 minutes. Add wine, peppercorns, and salt.

Debone the salmon (front two-thirds of fish) and remove any fat. Cut fish into 4 portions.

Return liquid to a low simmer, and slide in fish filets carefully. Turn heat to medium low to keep the liquid just below a simmer. Poaching liquid should just cover the salmon (add more water, if it does not). Cook fish gently, uncovered, 8–10 minutes. Lift pieces of fish from the liquid with a slotted spatula and transfer to a serving plate.

Make the salad: in a jar shake the balsamic vinegar and olive oil with a few pinches salt and pepper. Assemble all the prepared vegetables, dried fruit, and seeds; then dress the salad, to taste.

Serve with poached salmon overtop the salad, adding more dressing over the fish, as desired.

Shopping List

1 yellow beet
1 bunch parsley
2 lb. skinless wild salmon fillet
8 cups spinach greens

Check the Pantry

Balsamic vinegar
Bay leaves
Black peppercorns
Dried currants
Extra-virgin olive oil
Fennel seeds
Sea salt
Sunflower seeds
White wine

Saturday Dinner

Crab Cakes With Lemon "Aioli" and Kale With Caramelized Onions   Makes 10–12 cakes

Crab Cakes With Lemon "Aioli"

Additional Saturday dinner note to add: If you don't eat crab, you can use the same amount of raw salmon, by weight, and use a food processor to get an even consistency. Another alternative is to use cooked white beans in place of crab, mashing them up to make a paste before proceeding with the recipe.

Vegan variety: Use cooked white beans in place of crab for a delicious version.

Do ahead: Soak cashews overnight or a minimum of 4 hours.

½ cup lemon aioli (recipe follows)
½ bunch scallions, thinly sliced
¼ cup chopped onion
1 large egg, lightly beaten (or Ener-G Egg Replacer)
1 Tbsp. Dijon mustard
1 Tbsp. fresh lemon juice, plus wedges for garnish
½ cup celery, finely diced
3 Tbsp. homemade Old Bay seasoning (recipe below)
½ lb. fresh lump crab meat, picked over

½ cup of gluten-free bread crumbs (or 1 pack rice crackers, pulsed until breadcrumb-like)
¼ cup Bob's Red Mill All-Purpose, Gluten-Free Flour
2 Tbsp. extra-virgin olive oil
½ tsp. sea salt, or more to taste
¼ tsp. freshly ground black pepper, or more to taste
½ cup coconut oil, for frying

Whisk the first 8 ingredients in a bowl (lemon aioli through 3 tablespoons Old Bay seasoning). Add the crab, folding to blend. Add in the cracker crumbs, flour, olive oil, salt, and pepper. Divide crab mixture into 1-inch-thick patties (use a ¼ cup). Refrigerate for at least 40 minutes.

Heat ¼ cup coconut oil in a skillet on medium-high heat, adding enough oil to coat the bottom of the pan generously.

Fry cakes until golden brown, 3–4 minutes per side. Place cooked cakes on a baking sheet and keep warm in the oven on 350 degrees F until ready to serve. Serve with lemon wedges and more aioli (recipe below).

Homemade Old Bay Seasoning

2 tsp. celery salt
1 tsp. mustard powder
½ tsp. freshly ground black pepper
½ tsp. paprika
½ tsp. white pepper
½ tsp. ground ginger
¼ tsp. ground nutmeg

Combine all ingredients and mix until evenly blended.

Photo by Ben Garvey Photography

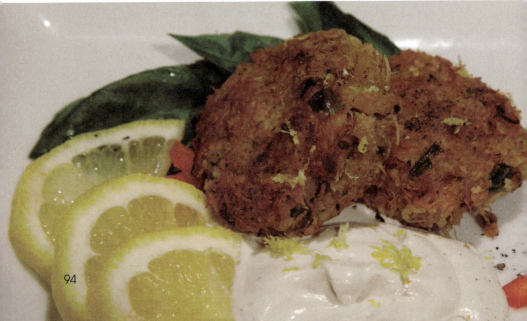

Lemon "Aioli" Makes 2 cups

2 cups cashews, soaked 4 hours or more
¼ cup lemon zest
3 Tbsp. lemon juice
3 cloves garlic, minced
¼ cup water
1 Tbsp. apple cider vinegar
½–1 tsp. sea salt, to taste

Combine ingredients in a high-speed blender and process until very smooth. Season to taste.

Shop List	Check the Pantry
2 cups raw unsalted cashew pieces	Apple cider vinegar
½ lb. fresh lump crabmeat, picked over	Black peppercorns
½ bunch celery	Celery salt
1 egg	Coconut oil
3 cloves garlic	Dijon mustard
1 lemon	Gluten-free all-purpose flour
1 bunch scallions	Gluten-free breadcrumbs or rice crackers
1 small yellow onion	Ground ginger
	Ground nutmeg
	Mustard powder
	Paprika
	Salt
	White pepper

Kale With Caramelized Onions Serves 4

¼ cup coconut oil
¼ cup extra-virgin olive oil
2 yellow onions, sliced
½ tsp. sea salt
2 bunches kale, destemmed and chopped

Heat the oil in a medium-size heavy skillet over medium-high heat. Add the sliced onion and the salt. Brown the onions for 5–7 minutes, stirring occasionally. Reduce heat to low and caramelize the onions for 20–30 minutes more, stirring occasionally. Add kale and ⅓ cup water. Bring heat to high and cover the skillet to steam the kale. Season with a few pinches of salt and pepper, to taste.

Sunday Brunch

Berry Green   Serves 1

The antioxidants in berries can help your body fight oxidative stress caused by free radicals. Eating a diet rich in antioxidants can help improve your health, protect your skin and hair, and fight inflammation.

1 green apple
½ lemon, peeled if not organic
1 cup berries, fresh or thawed if frozen
1 handful spinach
2 leaves kale
½ cucumber

Cut produce to fit your juicer's feed tube. Juice ½ apple and lemon. Turn off the machine and add the berries, then top with the plunger. Turn the machine back on and push berries through; add the greens, cucumber, and remaining apple. Stir the juice and pour into a glass; serve chilled.

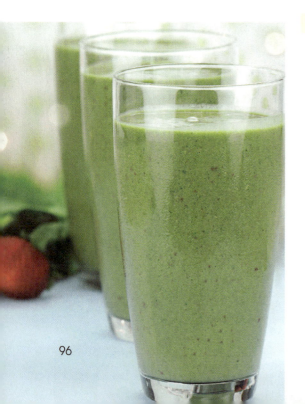

Spanish Frittata and Simple Salad With Maple Orange Vinaigrette Serves 4–6

Spanish Frittata

My mom used to make a Spanish tortilla (much like this recipe) almost every Sunday for lunch with a big fresh salad. I learned many great recipes from my mom, and this is one that I've adapted by removing the dairy. It is an easy one-dish meal. Thanks, Mom!

12 large organic eggs
½ cup coconut milk
½ tsp. sea salt, or more to taste
2 Tbsp. coconut oil or extra-virgin olive oil
1 small red onion, small chop
½ cup sautéed mushrooms or favorite vegetable of choice
1 cup spinach or arugula

Preheat the oven to 375 degrees.

In a medium bowl whisk the eggs and coconut milk with 2 pinches of salt. Set aside.

In a 4–6" skillet or omelet pan over medium-high heat add the coconut oil, red onion, and another pinch of salt. Sauté, stirring occasionally until the onion becomes translucent, about 3 minutes. Add the mushrooms or vegetables of choice and sauté until soft. Toss in spinach and fold into veggie mixture just until wilted. Remove the vegetables from pan. Set aside.

Turn down the heat to low, adding a little more coconut oil if needed. Using

Photo by Polara Studio

the same skillet, add the eggs, shaking to distribute the mixture evenly. Cook over medium-low heat for 5 minutes, using a spatula to spread the eggs from the edges to the center until the edges are no longer runny. Arrange the vegetable mixure over the top evenly.

Transfer to a 375-degree oven and cook for 5 minutes until set and slightly browned. Remove from oven. Be very aware of the hot handle!

To finish, slide partially cooked frittata onto a large plate; wearing oven mitts, place a plate over the pan and, holding the two together, invert them so the frittata drops onto the plate. Slide the frittata back into the pan so partially cooked side is up. Place back in oven to cook 3–4 minutes more.

Cut into wedges and serve.

Shopping List

1 dozen eggs
½ cup mushrooms
1 small red onion
2 cups spinach or arugula

Check the Pantry

Coconut milk
Coconut oil or extra-virgin olive oil
Sea salt

Simple Salad With Maple Orange Vinaigrette   Serves 4

This is a recipe I dreamed up for a "breakfast for dinner" themed night at our restaurant. Each week we serve four-course dinners, and we often choose an ethnic theme, preparing seasonal ingredients with a worldly twist. Breakfast for dinner was a departure from our normal menu set, as variety is the key of life. I love to teach this recipe for our brunch hands-on classes.

Vinaigrette Ingredients

½ cup extra-virgin olive oil
⅓–½ cup apple cider vinegar (adjust to taste)
⅓ cup maple syrup
1½ tsp. orange zest
Juice of 1 orange
1 tsp. fresh thyme, finely chopped
¾ tsp. sea salt
Freshly ground black pepper, to taste

In a bowl combine ingredients and whisk to combine well. Keep refrigerated and shake or whisk again before dressing your salad. Drizzle 4 large handfuls of salad greens with dressing just before serving and toss.

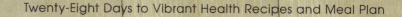

Shopping List

1 orange
4 large handfuls salad greens
   (one per person)
2 sprigs fresh thyme

Check the Pantry

Apple cider vinegar
Black peppercorns
Extra-virgin olive oil
Maple syrup
Sea salt

Sunday Dinner

Bay Leaf Roasted Chicken With Roasted Carrots and Kale With Fig Balsamic Dressing   Serves 4–6

Bay Leaf Roasted Chicken

Find fresh bay leaves in the refrigerated section of your store—they make this recipe! Crack them once to release the amazing aroma that seasons the chicken. I always season under the skin when roasting bone-in chicken.

3½–4 lb. chicken, free-range or organic
12 fresh bay leaves, cracked
4 cloves garlic, cut into coins
Sea salt
2 Tbsp. extra-virgin olive oil
Freshly ground black pepper
½ cup dry white wine

Preheat oven to 475 (your oven might smoke; be sure to turn the hood fan on!). Place rack in the middle of oven. Clean chicken (remove excess fat and giblets in cavity). Wash inside and out under cold water and pat dry with towel. Tuck wings back behind the first joints.

Use fingertips to loosen the skin from flesh, beginning at the breast and down to the thigh on each side.

Place 2 bay leaves in the cavity of the chicken. Insert remaining leaves under the skin, dispersing evenly along with the garlic coins. (2 per thigh, 3 per breast). Salt slightly under the skin. Tie legs with twine.

Place chicken breast side up in roasting pan. Rub olive oil over the skin and add salt and pepper. Roast 50–60 min-

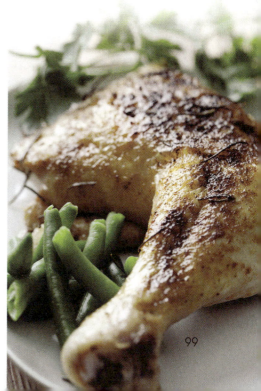

utes for whole bird, until skin is beautifully brown and juices run clear, not pink when cut into the leg. Be sure to baste the chicken once with the juices in the pan. Rest 10 minutes before cutting.

Optional: heat the juices in the pan on the stove, and add the white wine to create a quick jus for the chicken.

Shopping List	Check the Pantry
12 fresh bay leaves	Black peppercorns
1 whole chicken, free-range or organic	Extra-virgin olive oil or safflower oil
4 cloves garlic	Sea salt
	Dry white wine (optional)

Roasted Carrots   Serves 4

6 large carrots
½ tsp. sea salt
3 Tbsp. grape seed or coconut oil
¼ cup fresh herbs (tarragon, rosemary, etc.)

Preheat the oven to 400.

Place carrots in a pot and cover with water. Salt the water, turn on high heat and cover until the water starts to simmer. Simmer for 2 minutes, then strain.

Toss parboiled carrots in a bowl with oil, salt, and chopped fresh herb of choice. Spread out on a baking sheet.

Bake in the oven for 20–25 minutes or until golden brown and cooked through. Toss once during cook time to brown both sides.

Shopping List	Check the Pantry
5 carrots	Grape seed or coconut oil
¼ cup fresh herb of choice	Sea salt

Kale With Fig Balsamic Dressing   Serves 4

2 bunches lacinato or black kale, destemmed and roughly torn
2 Tbsp. extra-virgin olive oil
1–2 bunches turnip or radish greens (1–2 cups)
½ tsp. sea salt
¼ cup Fig Balsamic Dressing (Week One: Thursday Lunch)
½ cup unsweetened dried cranberries (optional)
Freshly ground black pepper, to taste

Heat a large skillet over medium-high heat. Once hot, add the olive oil then the kale and ½ of the salt to start. Using tongs, coat the greens with the oil until wilted. (Toss in the optional cranberries here.)

Add the Fig Balsamic Dressing, tossing gently to coat the greens. Taste, and season with more vinaigrette and/or salt, to taste.

Finish with cracked black pepper, to taste.

Shopping List

2 bunches lacinato kale
1–2 bunches turnip or radish
   tops

Check the Pantry

Balsamic vinegar
Black peppercorns
Dried cranberries
Extra-virgin olive oil
Sea salt

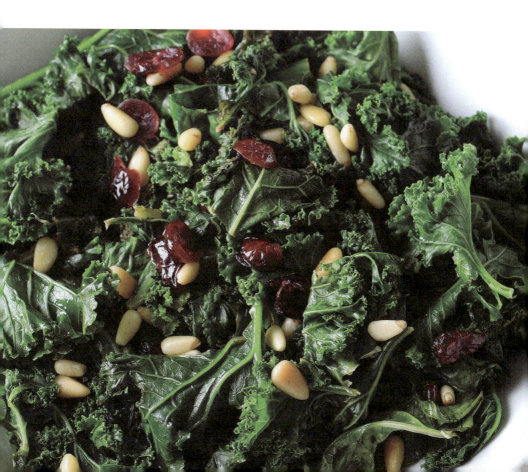

Week Two Shopping List

Cooking wine and vinegar

- ❏ 1 cup apple cider
- ❏ Apple cider vinegar
- ❏ Aged balsamic vinegar
- ❏ Red wine vinegar
- ❏ Rice vinegar
- ❏ Dry white wine (or more stock)

Dairy and eggs

- ❏ 10 large organic eggs

Dry herbs and spices

- ❏ Astralagus root (optional)
- ❏ Clove
- ❏ Cardamom pods
- ❏ Chili flakes (optional)
- ❏ Cinnamon stick
- ❏ Ginger powder
- ❏ Ground cardamom
- ❏ Ground cinnamon
- ❏ Ground coriander
- ❏ Ground cumin
- ❏ Ground turmeric
- ❏ Dried oregano

Dry or canned pantry items

- ❏ Almond extract
- ❏ Almond milk (8 oz.)
- ❏ Baking powder
- ❏ Gluten-free breadcrumbs or almond meal
- ❏ Chickpea miso
- ❏ Coconut aminos or tamari
- ❏ 2 cans coconut milk (15 oz.)
- ❏ Coconut sugar
- ❏ Dijon mustard
- ❏ Fish sauce or umeboshi vinegar
- ❏ Raw honey
- ❏ Maple syrup or date syrup
- ❏ Sea salt
- ❏ Liquid stevia (suggest Sweet Leaf Vanilla Creme)
- ❏ Vanilla extract
- ❏ Wasabi powder

Flours

- ❏ Arrowroot/tapioca flour

- ❏ Gluten-free all-purpose flour
- ❏ ¾ tsp. xanthum gum

Fresh herbs and spices

- ❏ 1 bunch basil
- ❏ 3 bunches cilantro
- ❏ 11 inches ginger
- ❏ 2 Tbsp. fresh lavender (optional)
- ❏ 3 bunches mint
- ❏ 2 bunches parsley
- ❏ 2 sprigs rosemary

Fish, poultry, meat

- ❏ 6 whole chicken legs, free-range
- ❏ 5 chicken thighs or breasts, boneless
- ❏ 1½ lb. boneless chicken
- ❏ 1½ lb. rockfish
- ❏ 1½–2 lb. wild salmon
- ❏ 1½ lb. wild shrimp, peeled and deveined (or chicken)

Grains and beans

- ❏ 1 cup black beans
- ❏ 2 cups dried chickpeas
- ❏ 3 cups quinoa

- ❏ 1 cup brown rice
- ❏ 2 packages thin rice noodles

Nuts and seeds

- ❏ 2 cups almond milk or coconut milk
- ❏ 1 cup cashews
- ❏ Shredded coconut flakes
- ❏ ½ cup hazelnuts
- ❏ ½ cup pumpkin seeds
- ❏ 3 cups walnuts

Oils

- ❏ Coconut oil
- ❏ Extra-virgin olive oil
- ❏ Grape seed oil
- ❏ Unrefined sesame oil

Produce

Fruit

- ❏ 7 apples
- ❏ 1 green apple
- ❏ 3 avocados
- ❏ 6 lemons
- ❏ 7 limes
- ❏ 1 mango
- ❏ 1 papaya
- ❏ 2 pears

❏ Fresh or frozen pineapple (enough for ½ cup)

❏ ½ pint strawberries

❏ 2 lb. stone fruit (plums, nectarines, peaches)

Stocks

❏ 3 quarts chicken stock

❏ 2 quarts vegetable stock

Vegetables

❏ 2 bunches asparagus

❏ 5 cups arugula or watercress (¼–½ lb.)

❏ Baby spinach to equal 3 cups

❏ 1 beet

❏ 1 head bok coy

❏ 1 head broccoli

❏ 3 lb. butternut squash

❏ 6½ lb. carrots

❏ ½ head celery

❏ 1 head collard greens

❏ 4 cucumbers

❏ 1 English (seedless) cucumber

❏ 1½ head fennel

❏ 2 heads garlic

❏ 2 cups green beans

❏ 1 small green cabbage

❏ 2 bunches kale

❏ 1 pint mung bean sprouts

❏ 2 bunches mustard greens

❏ 1 small red onion

❏ 2 heads romaine lettuce (or greens of choice)

❏ 4 cups mixed salad greens (¼ lb.)

❏ 3 bunches scallions

❏ 2 shallots

❏ 1 cup shiitake mushrooms (optional)

❏ 1 pint sprouts of choice

❏ 2 lb. sweet potatoes

❏ 2 lb. root vegetables (parsnips, rutabaga)

❏ 3 lb. yellow onion

Your choice DIY salad vegetables (8 cups total needed):

❏ Arugula

❏ Asparagus

❏ Beets

❏ Bok choy

❏ Carrots

❏ Celery

❏ Cooked beans

❏ Daikon

- ❏ Dandelion greens
- ❏ Fava beans
- ❏ Jicama
- ❏ Mustard greens
- ❏ Nectarines
- ❏ Peaches
- ❏ Pears
- ❏ Radicchio
- ❏ Radish
- ❏ Scallions
- ❏ Strawberries
- ❏ Swiss chard
- ❏ Turnip
- ❏ Watercress

Week Two Menu and Recipes

Monday Breakfast

On the Green   Serves 1–2

Parsley contains myristicin, a volatile oil that has been shown to activate the enzyme glutathione S-transferase (GST). This enzyme helps to deactivate molecules that would otherwise damage the body. The unique oils in parsley make it a "chemoprotective" food, meaning a food that can help neutralize particular types of carcinogens that can cause cancer.

1 cucumber, peeled if not organic and chopped
½ cup chopped kale
½ cup chopped parsley
½ cup frozen pineapple pieces
1 Tbsp. organic virgin coconut oil
6–8 ice cubes

Combine all ingredients in a blender and process until smooth and creamy. Pour into a glass and serve chilled.

Shopping List

1 cucumber
1 bunch kale
1 bunch parsley
1 small fresh pineapple or 1 bag
   frozen pineapple pieces

Check the Pantry

Virgin coconut oil

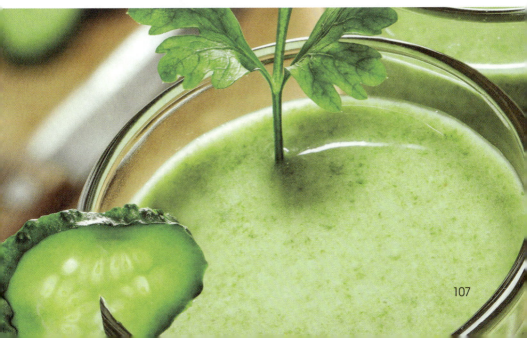

Monday Lunch

Asparagus Ribbon Salad With Sliced Chicken   Serves 4

Asparagus is high in B vitamins and helps balance healthy blood sugar levels. Watercress and arugula are pungent greens and help expel toxins from the body. This is a healthy, pretty salad that is worth the effort of peeling the asparagus into ribbons. Add edible flowers if you can find them.

1 bunch fresh asparagus, rinsed, stems and tips removed
3 cups arugula or watercress
1 shallot, minced
¼ cup freshly squeezed lemon juice
¼ cup extra-virgin olive oil
2 cooked chicken breasts, sliced
2 Tbsp. honey
Sea salt
Freshly ground black pepper
¼ cup hazelnuts, roasted and roughly chopped

Rinse vegetables. Chop shallot and set aside. Squeeze fresh lemon juice. Snap off asparagus ends. Use a peeler to shave asparagus into ribbons. Lay asparagus spears flat and peel, flipping when one side gets too thin. Repeat. Snap last thin pieces of asparagus in half and add to salad. Set asparagus aside in a bowl.

Dressing

Whisk lemon juice, honey, and shallot in a bowl. Drizzle in olive oil and whisk constantly. Add salt and pepper, to taste. Toss asparagus with dressing to coat. Let rest 15 minutes.

Toast hazelnuts in a pan until fragrant. Add arugula/watercress and chicken to marinated asparagus, and season to taste. Plate salad with layers of toasted hazelnuts. Top with fresh pepper.

Shopping List	Check the Pantry
1 bunch fresh asparagus	Black peppercorns
3 cups arugula or watercress	Extra-virgin olive oil
1 lemon	Raw honey
¼ cup hazelnuts	Sea salt
1 shallot	

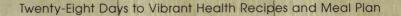

Monday Dinner

Herb and Chickpea Croquettes With Rosemary Walnut Pesto and Cider-Braised Greens and Green Beans
Serves 4

Herb and Chickpea Croquettes

1½ cup chickpeas, cooked
⅓ cup extra-virgin olive oil, for batter
1 cup cooked quinoa
½ cup shallot, diced
2 garlic cloves, minced
½ cup celery, diced
½ tsp. dried oregano
½ tsp. sea salt
1 Tbsp. Dijon mustard
1¼ cup almond meal or gluten-free breadcrumbs
⅓ cup all-purpose gluten-free flour
Coconut or grape seed oil, for pan frying

Pulse the chickpeas and olive oil together in food processor, or mash in a bowl with a tool. Combine all ingredients in a bowl and add the mashed chickpeas and oil. Taste for flavor and let sit 10 minutes. If dough seems dry, add more olive oil until you can easily form a ball in your hand. Form into balls no bigger than 2 inches in diameter.

Heat a pan with ¼ cup coconut oil over medium-high heat until very hot. Fry croquettes 2 minutes per side, and if needed place on a baking sheet and finish cooking in the oven on 350 degrees until browned and crispy on the exterior but not dry, about 5–10 minutes.

Replenish oil as needed, changing out oil if brown bits form (scrape oil into a bowl lined with a strainer so you can use the oil once more for pan frying).

Shopping List	Check the Pantry
½ cup celery	Chickpeas
2 cloves garlic	Coconut or grape seed oil
½ cup shallots	Dijon mustard
	Dried oregano
	Extra-virgin olive oil
	Gluten-free flour all-purpose flour
	Gluten-free breadcrumbs or almond meal
	Quinoa
	Sea salt

Rosemary Walnut Pesto   Yields 2 cups

Pesto in our kitchen takes on many forms through the seasons. This is a winter pesto recipe we love—try it with kale in place of parsley! Come summer, substitute basil or cilantro for the rosemary (about ½ cup) to keep this recipe current with the season.

1 bunch parsley
2 sprigs rosemary
1 clove garlic
1 cup walnut
⅓ cup chickpeas or white miso
¾ tsp. sea salt, to taste
1 cup extra-virgin olive oil

Combine the first 6 ingredients in a food processor, slowly pouring in the olive oil. Adjust flavor and consistency as desired. Add the juice of half a lemon for a bonus alkalizing kick!

Shopping List	Check the Pantry
1 clove garlic	Chickpeas or white miso
1 bunch parsley	Extra-virgin olive oil
2 sprigs rosemary	Hazelnut
	Sea salt

Cider-Braised Greens and Green Beans   Serves 4

1 cup apple cider
¼ cup coconut oil
1 tsp. sea salt
1 head collard greens, destemmed and chopped
2 cups green beans, destemmed and chopped
1 Tbsp. apple cider vinegar

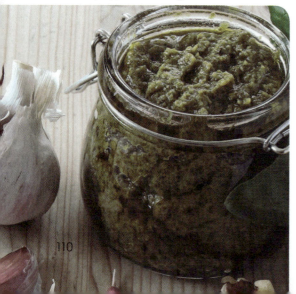

Heat apple cider in a medium size skillet over high heat. Allow the cider to reduce at a rapid boil for 5 minutes, or until reduced by half.

Add oil and salt and stir to combine. Add collard greens, green beans, and apple cider vinegar and continue to boil.

Lower heat to low and braise for 5–7 minutes. Taste and serve.

Shopping List

1 cup apple cider
1 head collard greens
2 cups green beans

Check the Pantry

Apple cider vinegar
Coconut oil
Sea salt

Tuesday Breakfast

Morning Energy   Serves 1–2

Beets contain unique phytonutrients called betalains, which have been shown to provide antioxidant, anti-inflammatory, and detoxification effects.

1–2 carrots, scrubbed well, tops removed, ends trimmed
½ small beet, with leaves
1 cucumber, peeled if not organic
1 handful spinach or several chard leaves
½ lemon, peeled
1-inch-piece ginger root, scrubbed, peeled if old

Cut produce to fit your juicer's feed tube. Juice all ingredients and stir. Pour into a glass and drink as soon as possible.

Shopping List

1 cup baby spinach or 1 bunch
    chard
1 beet with leaves
1–2 carrots
1 cucumber
1-inch-piece ginger root
1 lemon

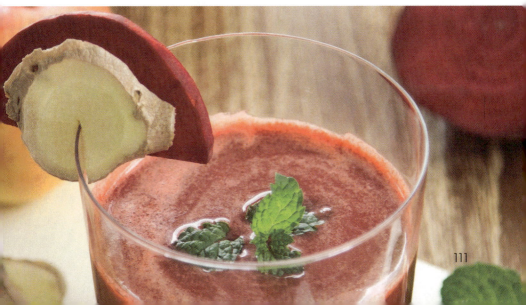

Easy Omelet With Greens and Basil   Serves 4

Here is a great way to practice omelet making. Make sure to keep the heat on medium and lower the heat if the eggs start to brown. Rolling the omelets make them especially fancy. However fancy, they are easy to make!

8 large organic eggs
¼ tsp. sea salt
2 Tbsp. extra-virgin olive oil
2 large handful chopped arugula or spinach
½ cup basil leaves
1½ Tbsp. aged balsamic vinegar
Freshly ground black pepper, to taste

Preheat oven to 300 degrees.

Note: You will do this whole process twice to yield 2 large omelets to cut in half, for 4 servings. If your pan is small, repeat 4 times, making 1 omelet per person.

Beat the eggs and salt in a small bowl, until eggs are a uniform color.

Heat a medium-large sized nonstick pan over medium heat. Brush lightly with olive oil, and pour in half of the egg mixture (for 2 large omelets, or ¼ of the egg mixture for 4 omelets).

Swirl the pan so the egg spreads out evenly across the pan in a very thin layer. Let set (2–3 minutes). Run a spatula underneath the omelet and slide it out of the pan onto a lined baking sheet.

Add greens and basil to the inside of the omelet and roll away from you. Cut in half and warm slightly in the oven to wilt the greens and cook the egg in the center.

Finish with a drizzle of balsamic vinegar or pepper, to taste.

Shopping List

2 large handful chopped
    arugula or spinach
½ cup basil leaves
8 large organic eggs

Check the Pantry

Aged balsamic vinegar (optional)
Black peppercorns
Extra-virgin olive oil
Sea salt

Tuesday Lunch

Tropical Quinoa Salad With Cashews With Carrot Fries
Serves 4

Tropical Quinoa Salad

1 cup dried quinoa, rinsed well
½ red onion, finely chopped
1 cup apple or carrot, finely chopped
Juice of 1 lime
2 tsp. honey or agave
1 Tbsp. extra-virgin olive oil
1 large mango, chopped *(not overly ripe)*
¼ cup mint, finely chopped
½ cup cilantro, finely chopped
1 tsp. sea salt, to taste
Freshly ground black pepper, to taste
½-inch-piece ginger, finely chopped
1 avocado, chopped or thinly sliced
1 cup cashews, coarsely chopped
3 cups Romaine lettuce (or greens of choice), roughly chopped

Cook the quinoa: Bring 2 cups of water to a boil in a medium saucepan, add the quinoa, and simmer, covered for 15–20 minutes. Set aside and let cool (spread out for best results).

In a large bowl toss the chopped red onion and apple/carrot. Whisk together the lime juice, honey, and olive oil. Add to the bowl. Add the cooked, cooled quinoa and mango to the bowl and toss well. Mix in mint, cilantro, ginger, and salt and pepper, to taste.

Garnish with sliced avocado and cashews. Scoop mixture over greens and serve chilled or at room temperature.

Photo by Polara Studio

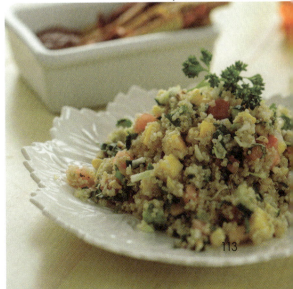

Carrot Fries   Serves 4

Here is a lovely alternative to the potato fry. Who doesn't like french fries? Really. There are many root vegetable alternatives to the "french fry" that are better for the body and don't contribute to inflammation like potatoes. So, behold! A fun baked fry recipe: try it with parsnips or rutabaga, or even beets!

2 large handfuls of carrots (8 or so)
3 Tbsp. grape seed oil (plus more for the pan)
2 tsp. ground turmeric
Few pinches of sea salt

Preheat the oven to 425 degrees and oil a baking sheet. Slice the carrots into ¼-inch strips (think french fries). In a large bowl toss the carrots with oil, turmeric, and salt.

Line the fries in a single layer on an oiled baking sheet and bake until golden brown, about 12–15 minutes, turning twice. Be sure to give the fries room (move to two sheets if you made a lot)

Remove from oven, let cool, and enjoy. Try not to eat them all off the pan!

Shopping List

1 apple or ½ pint of strawberries (choose what's in season)
1 avocado
8 carrots
1 bunch cilantro
1 lime
1 mango
1 bunch mint
1 small red onion
1 head romaine lettuce (or green of choice)

Check the Pantry

Black peppercorns
Cashews
Extra-virgin olive oil
Grape seed oil
Ground turmeric
Quinoa
Raw honey
Sea salt

Tuesday Dinner

Roasted Chicken Legs With Roasted Sweet Potatoes and a Simple Salad With Dijon Dressing   Serves 4–6

Roasted Chicken Legs

6 whole chicken legs (thigh and leg), free-range
4 cloves garlic, cut into coins
2 Tbsp. grape seed oil
Sea salt
Freshly ground black pepper
½ cup dry white wine

Preheat oven to 475. Place rack in the middle of oven. Clean chicken (remove excess fat). Wash inside and out under cold water and pat dry with towel.

Use fingertips to loosen the skin from flesh, and tuck the garlic beneath the skin—try not to break the skin as you do this.

Place chicken in roasting pan. Rub oil over the skin and generously sprinkle with salt and pepper. Roast for 30 minutes, until skin is beautifully brown and juices run clear, not pink when cut into the leg. Rest 10 minutes before cutting to serve.

Optional: heat the remaining juices left in the pan on the stove, and add the white wine to create a quick sauce for the chicken.

Shopping List

6 whole chicken legs, free-range
4 cloves garlic

Check the Pantry

Black peppercorns
Dry white wine (optional)
Grape seed oil
Sea salt

Roasted Sweet Potatoes

2 large sweet potatoes
3 Tbsp. sunflower or grape seed oil
½ tsp. sea salt

Preheat the oven to 400.

Cut the sweet potatoes in long wedge pieces about 1–2 inches thick. Toss the wedges in a bowl with oil and salt, and then spread out on a baking sheet. Bake in the oven for 30–35 minutes, or until golden brown. Toss once during cook time to brown both sides.

Shopping List

2 large sweet potatoes

Check the Pantry

Sea salt
Sunflower or grape seed oil

Simple Salad With Dijon Dressing

2 Tbsp. Dijon mustard
3 Tbsp. apple cider vinegar
⅓ cup extra-virgin olive oil
4 handfuls mixed salad greens
½ cup pumpkin seeds
Sea salt, to taste
Freshly ground black pepper, to taste

Combine Dijon mustard, vinegar, and oil in a jar and shake until combined. Toss with salad greens and pumpkin seeds in a bowl, adding salt and pepper, to taste.

Shopping List

4 handfuls mixed salad greens

Check the Pantry

Apple cider vinegar
Black peppercorns
Dijon mustard
Extra-virgin olive oil
Pumpkin seeds
Sea salt

Wednesday Breakfast

Papaya Dreamsicle   Serves 1

Papaya has the unique protein-digesting enzymes papain and chymopapain, which have been shown to help lower inflammation.

1 cup unsweetened almond milk
1 papaya, cut into pieces and frozen (about 1½ cups)
½ cup chopped flat-leaf parsley
1½ tsp. organic lemon peel, freshly grated
1 tsp. pure vanilla extract

Place all ingredients in a blender and process until smooth and creamy. Pour into glass and serve chilled.

Shopping List

1 container unsweetened
   almond milk
1 bunch flat leaf parsley
1 lemon
1 papaya

Check the Pantry

Pure vanilla extract

Wednesday Lunch

Sesame Kale Salad With Apple With Butternut Squash Bisque   Serves 4–6

Sesame Kale Salad With Apple

2 cups apple, sliced or shredded
1 clove garlic, minced
6 cups kale, chopped into bite-size pieces
1-inch-piece of ginger, minced (optional)
1 tsp. sea salt
2 Tbsp. lemon juice
1 Tbsp. extra-virgin olive oil
½ Tbsp. sesame oil

Combine all ingredients in a large bowl. With clean hands massage the vegetables as if you are squeezing water out of them. Work the vegetables at least 15 times.

After 10 minutes, use a plate to hold the vegetables in the bowl, and tilt to drain the excess liquid into the sink. Work the vegetables another 15 times.

If you prefer a saltier or more pickled salad repeat the process 1–2 more times. Enjoy many variations on the theme!

Shopping List	Check the Pantry
2 apples	Extra-virgin olive oil
1 clove garlic	Sea salt
1-inch-piece ginger	Sesame oil
2 bunches kale	
1 lemon	

Butternut Squash Bisque   Serves 8

3 lb. carrots or yams, peeled
   and cut into ¾-inch pieces
3 lb. butternut squash, peeled,
   seeded, and diced
2 lb. yellow onion, chopped
2 Tbsp. grape seed oil
Sea salt, to taste
Freshly ground black pepper,
   to taste
6 cups vegetable broth
1 cup coconut milk
1 tsp. ground cardamom (or
   cinnamon)

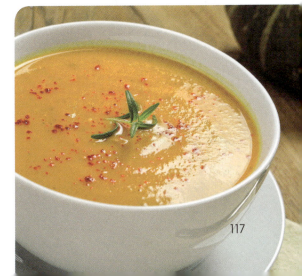

Preheat oven to 425 degrees. Toss carrots, squash, and onions in oil and spread vegetables onto a large lined baking sheet (or two small sheets). Season with salt and pepper, then roast for 20 minutes until tender, stirring once or twice.

Remove from the oven and transfer directly to a pot. Add broth, coconut milk and cardamom/cinnamon. Simmer for 10 minutes.

Carefully working in batches, puree the soup in a blender or food processor until smooth and season to taste with salt until desired flavor is reached.

Three variation ideas: Add ½ cup apple cider. Add ¼ cup lemon juice. Add ¼ cup lime juice.

Shopping List

3 lb. butternut squash
3 lb. carrots
2 lb. yellow onions (about two)

Check the Pantry

Black peppercorns
Coconut milk
Grape seed oil
Ground cardamom or cinnamon
Sea salt
Vegetable stock

Wednesday Dinner

Stir-Fry Rockfish and Mustard Greens Over Mashed Sweet Potatoes   Serves 4

Stir-Fry Rockfish and Mustard Greens

1½ lb. rockfish, cut into 1–1½-inch pieces
2-inch-piece ginger, minced
2 cloves garlic, minced
1 Tbsp. fish sauce or umeboshi vinegar
½ cup shredded coconut flakes (optional)
2 cups mustard greens, chiffonade
2 Tbsp. coconut oil for frying
1 bunch scallions, thinly sliced
½ tsp. sea salt, to taste
2 Tbsp. tamari or coconut aminos
2 Tbsp. lime juice
½ cup cilantro, chopped
¼ cup mint, chopped

Marinate the fish with minced ginger, minced garlic, fish sauce, and optional coconut flakes, tossing to coat evenly. Let sit 20 minutes. Place mustard greens in a bowl and set aside.

Heat coconut oil in a wok until very hot; add scallions and a pinch of salt, shaking pan to cook evenly. Brown scallions well and remove them from pan. Add fish to the pan and do not touch for 2 minutes.

Shake the pan and flip fish carefully (*no tongs!*) to cook evenly, adding tamari and lime juice. Cook 2–4 minutes more or until just done. Remove from pan and place in the bowl of chiffonade mustard greens, tossing to combine and wilt the greens slightly.

Stir in cilantro and mint to the stir-fry mixture, and add fried scallions as garnish to the salad. Serve with a squeeze of lime.

Serve over roasted or mashed sweet potatoes.

Shopping List

1 bunch cilantro
2 cloves garlic
2 inch ginger
2 Tbsp. lime juice
¼ cup mint
1 bunch mustard greens
1½ lb. rockfish
1 bunch scallions

Check the Pantry

Coconut oil
Fish sauce or umeboshi vinegar
Sea salt
Shredded coconut flakes
Tamari or coconut aminos

Roasted Sweet Potatoes (see Week Two: Tuesday Dinner) or Mashed Sweet Potatoes   Serves 4

2 lb. sweet potatoes
¼ cup extra-virgin olive oil
¾ tsp. sea salt, or more to taste
¼ cup coconut milk
Freshly ground black pepper

Peel the potatoes and cut them into medium-size pieces. Put them in a large (4 quart) saucepan, filling the pan with cold water. Cover the vegetables by 2 inches.

Bring the vegetables to a boil, covered, over high heat. Continue to boil until they are easily pierced with a fork, about 15–20 minutes. Drain and set aside.

In a large bowl toss the vegetables with olive and coconut oil, coconut milk, and salt. Mash with a potato masher until creamy, adding more salt if desired.

Do ahead option: keep the mashed veggies warm by keeping them in a covered metal bowl set over a pan of simmering water for up to an hour (double boiler).

Shopping List

2 lb. sweet potatoes

Check the Pantry

Black peppercorns
Coconut milk
Extra-virgin olive oil
Sea salt

Thursday Breakfast

You Are Loved Cocktail   Serves 1–2

Celery is a good source of vitamin C, beta-carotene, and manganese—antioxidants that have been shown to provide anti-inflammatory benefits.

3 carrots, scrubbed well, tops removed, ends trimmed
2 celery ribs with leaves
1 cucumber, peeled if not organic
1 handful spinach
1 lemon, peeled if not organic
½ beet, scrubbed well, with stems and leaves

Cut produce to fit your juicer's feed tube. Juice all ingredients and stir. Pour into a glass and drink as soon as possible.

Shopping List

1 beet with leaves
3 carrots
2 ribs celery
1 cucumber
1 lemon
1 handful spinach

Thursday Lunch

DIY Salad With Avocado and Chickpeas

DIY means "do it yourself." This is where the magic of salads happen: improvising in your kitchen with the produce you have, to make an on-the-fly fresh salad as a stand-alone meal or a side dish. Think outside of the lettuce box—chop up anything colorful and fresh for your salad, and experiment with fresh herbs to really brighten things up. Chop vegetables in bite-size pieces, especially if they are sturdy vegetables such as beets or carrots. Anchor your salad with avocado and chickpeas today to make it a meal in one.

Here is a starter list of ingredients for salad making. I encourage you to find even more ingredients to make your salads magical!

Apples
Arugula
Asparagus
Avocado
Cooked beans
Beets
Bok choy
Carrots
Celery
Cooked chickpeas
Daikon
Dandelion greens
Fava beans
Garlic
Ginger
Fresh herbs (basil, mint, cilantro,

rosemary)
Jicama
Kale Mustard greens
Nectarines
Nuts/seeds
Peaches
Pears
Radicchio
Radish
Scallions
Strawberries
Swiss chard
Turnips
Watercress

Shopping List

Your choice from the above list,
about 2–3 cups per person

Photo by Polara Studio

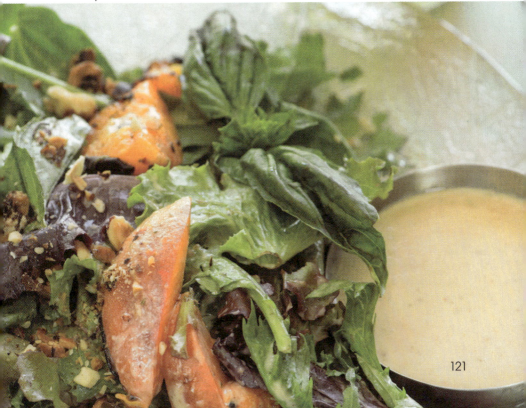

Thursday Dinner

Basil Stir-Fry With Chicken   Serves 4

Served with Basic Quinoa (Week One: Monday Lunch)

Fresh basil leaves make this recipe fresh and colorful. Use whole mint for a fun variation.

1 lb. boneless chicken (or tofu)
2 Tbsp. grape seed oil or coconut oil
1-inch-piece minced ginger
2 cloves minced garlic
2 cups carrots, sliced on the bias
1 head broccoli, cut into florets
1 head bok choy, sliced on the bias
½ cup whole basil leaves, packed (large stems removed)
4 Tbsp. stock (chicken) or water

Marinade

1–2 Tbsp. tamari (or coconut aminos)
1 Tbsp. arrowroot (or tapioca flour)
2 Tbsp. rice vinegar

Cut chicken into 2-inch pieces less than ½ inch wide. Mix the marinade in a bowl with a whisk to blend. Marinate the chicken for 10–20 minutes.

Heat the oil in a large skillet or a wok over very high heat. When the oil begins to ripple, stir in the meat, leaving marinade in the bowl for later use. When meat begins to brown add the garlic and ginger for 15 seconds, then add the vegetables.

Quickly stir the vegetables and chicken until both are done, about 3–5 minutes only. Stir in the stock or water and remaining marinade. Simmer for 1–2 minutes more.

Optional add-ins: 1 tsp. sesame oil, 2 Tbsp. agave nectar, 2 Tbsp. rice vinegar, 1 Tbsp. hot chile oil, ¼ cup cashews.

Shopping List	Check the Pantry
Basil	Arrowroot or tapioca flour
1 head bok choy	Chicken stock
1½ lb. boneless chicken	Coconut aminos or tamari
Broccoli	Coconut oil
6 carrots	Mirin or rice wine
Garlic	Quinoa
Ginger	
Scallions	

Friday Breakfast

Coconut Shake   Serves 1–2

In scientific studies coconut oil has been found to have anti-inflammatory and analgesic properties.

1 cup coconut milk
1 Tbsp. virgin coconut oil
1 Tbsp. ground flaxseeds
1 tsp. pure vanilla extract
¼ tsp. almond extract
Several drops of liquid stevia
8–10 ice cubes

Place all ingredients but ice in a blender and process at high speed until well combined. Add ice after the coconut oil is blended so that it won't clump. You may use more or less ice, depending on how cold you like a smoothie.

Shopping List	Check the Pantry
1 container or can coconut milk	Almond extract
1 package flaxseeds	Liquid stevia
	Pure vanilla extract
	Virgin coconut oil

Friday Lunch

Butternut Squash Bisque With DIY Salad

Treat yourself to your efforts this week! Thaw your soup and make a new version of a DIY salad with the ingredients you have on hand. This time-saving combo will set you up to enjoy a great weekend of new recipes ahead!

Butternut Squash Bisque—Week Two: Wednesday Lunch

DIY Salad—Week Two: Thursday Lunch

Friday Dinner

Asian Noodle Salad With Wild Shrimp With Lime Wasabi Vinaigrette Serves 4–6

Asian Noodle Salad With Wild Shrimp

½ lb. rice noodles
1½ lb. wild shrimp, peeled and deveined
2 Tbsp. sesame oil
4 carrots, shredded
1 English (seedless) cucumber, deseeded and shredded
2 cups mung bean sprouts, rinsed and drained
1 bunch scallions, thinly sliced
½ bunch greens of choice (mustard, bok choy, etc.)
2 cups toasted walnuts
¼ cup fresh cilantro or mint, coarsely chopped

Lime Wasabi Vinaigrette

2 Tbsp. wasabi powder (prepared with 2 Tbsp. warm water, resting 10 minutes before using)
½ cup lime juice
⅓ cup extra-virgin olive oil
½ tsp. sea salt
1½-inch-piece ginger, peeled and chopped
1 Tbsp. sesame oil

Photo by Polara Studio

Blend the vinaigrette ingredients, and set aside in a bowl.

Boil water in a stockpot and submerge the noodles. Turn off the heat and soften the noodles for 10 minutes.

Cook the shrimp in a medium skillet by adding ½ cup water to the pan. Bring to a boil, add the shrimp and cover until opaque and cooked through, about 5–6 minutes.

Drain noodles and place in a bowl with remaining ingredients. Add ½ cup Lime Wasabi Vinaigrette, to coat well, adding more to taste. Arrange the shrimp over the noodles, or toss all together.

This dish is great served at room temperature or chilled, with extra sauce on the side.

Shopping List

4 carrots
1 English (seedless) cucumber
1 bunch greens of choice
½ cup lime juice
1 bunch fresh mint or cilantro
2 cups mung bean sprouts
1 bunch scallions
1½ lb. wild shrimp, peeled and deveined

Check the Pantry

Extra-virgin olive oil
Rice noodles
Sea salt
Sesame oil
Walnuts, toasted
Wasabi powder

Saturday Breakfast

Mint Refresher   Serves 1–2

Fennel is rich in the phytonutrient anethole. In animal studies this nutrient has repeatedly been shown to reduce inflammation and to help prevent the occurrence of cancer.

2 stalks fennel with leaves
½ cucumber, peeled if not organic
½ green apple such as Granny Smith or pippin
1 small handful mint
1-inch-piece ginger root, scrubbed or peeled if old

Cut produce to fit your juicer's feed tube. Juice ingredients and stir. Pour into a glass and drink as soon as possible.

Shopping List

1 cucumber
1 fennel bulb
1-inch-piece of ginger root
1 green apple
1 bunch of mint

Saturday Lunch

All-Vegetable Spring Rolls With Ginger Mint Sauce
Serves 4

All-Vegetable Spring Rolls

These salad rolls with make you want to move. Ginger, mint, and mustard greens are all stimulating to the body, and help with focus and digestion. Pears nourish the lungs and also help move excess mucus or phlegm from the body. Get outdoors and play!

½ bunch mustard greens
½ bunch lettuce
1 shredded carrot
1 sliced pear
1 bunch scallions
1 avocado
½ cup sprouts
½ bunch cilantro
½ bunch basil
Cooked rice noodles (optional)
Shiitake mushrooms (optional)
Rice paper (large rounds)

Ginger Mint Sauce

¼ cup mint, finely chopped
3 Tbsp. ginger, minced
½ cup rice vinegar
⅓ cup extra-virgin olive oil

1 heaping Tbsp. honey
2 pinches sea salt
2 dried Thai chilies, sliced
  (optional)

Photo by Polara Studio

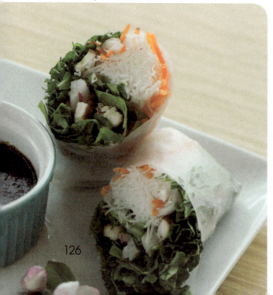

Combine all ingredients, whisk together, and set aside.

For the spring rolls: Gather your ingredients. Clean your produce well. Destem greens and lettuce. Shred the carrot. Slice the pear and scallions thinly. Slice the avocado. Get ready to roll.

Fill a large bowl with warm water. Dip the rice paper in warm water and swirl, 10 seconds.

Place a piece of rice paper on the cutting board, rough side down. Top with mustard greens, lettuce, and optional noodles and mushrooms. Line a bit of each remaining ingredient in the lower third of the wrap. Fold the side closest to you over the ingredients, then fold in both sides. Roll forward to complete and lay seam side down. Repeat until all ingredients are utilized. Then plate and serve with Ginger Mint Sauce.

Shopping List

1 avocado
1 bunch each basil, cilantro, and
   mint
1 carrot
1-inch ginger
1 head lettuce
1 bunch mustard greens
1 pear
1 pack rice paper wrappers
1 bunch scallions
1 cup shiitake mushrooms
   (optional)
1 pint sprouts
2 Thai chilies (dried, optional)

Check the Pantry

Extra-virgin olive oil
Raw honey
Rice noodles (vermicelli)
Rice vinegar
Sea salt

Saturday Dinner

Grilled Salmon and Asparaugs With Stone Fruit and Lavender Chutney   Serves 4–6

Think ripe peaches, plums, and nectarines. Think grilling. Think summer! This is a summer recipe through and through and is best enjoyed outside. I add a touch of lavender to the chutney for fun, but it's not essential.

Grilled Salmon and Asparagus

1½–2 lb. wild salmon
2 bunches asparagus
2 Tbsp. extra-virgin olive oil
Sea salt, to taste
Freshly ground black pepper, to taste

Prepare the grill for high heat.
   Brush the salmon with olive oil on both sides. Salt and pepper salmon liberally.
   Lightly oil the asparagus and season with salt and pepper. Place asparagus on the grill and grill for 5–7 minutes or until bright green and glistening.
   Grill the salmon skin side down for 5 minutes. Flip and continue cooking 4–5 minutes or until cooked. Remove salmon from the grill and top with chutney.

Stone Fruit and Lavender Chutney

2 lb. stone fruit, small dice
1 large onion, finely chopped
Zest of 1 lemon or lime
2 Tbsp. garlic, minced
¼ tsp. chili flakes (optional)
⅓ cup red wine vinegar
¾ cup raw honey or agave
¾ tsp. sea salt
2 Tbsp. fresh lavender (or use basil or mint; use only 1 tsp. dried lavender if you cannot find it fresh)

In a saucepan combine all prepared ingredients expect the herbs. Bring to a boil. Continue cooking at a rolling boil, 15 minutes. Stir occasionally. Mix in fresh herbs and/or lavender at the end.

Shopping List	Check the Pantry
2 bunches asparagus	Black peppercorns
2 cloves garlic	Chili flakes (optional)
2 Tbsp. fresh lavender, basil, or mint	Extra-virgin olive oil
1 lemon or lime	Raw honey or agave
1½–2 lb. wild salmon	Red wine vinegar
2 lb. stone fruit	Sea salt
1 yellow onion	

Photo by Polara Studio

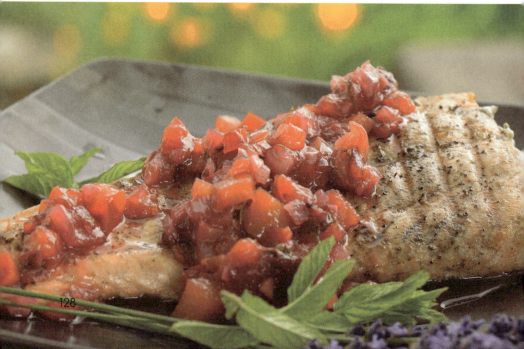

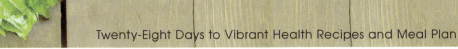

Sunday Breakfast

Sweet Green Chai   Serves 2

Spinach contains alpha-lipoic acid, which helps vitamins C and E regenerate and
has anti-inflammatory effects.

1 cup almond milk
1 pear, cut into pieces
1 cup baby spinach
½ tsp. ground cinnamon
⅛ tsp. ground cardamom
⅛ tsp. ground coriander
⅛ tsp. ground cloves
⅛ tsp. freshly ground black pepper
5–6 drops stevia
6 ice cubes (or 6 cubes of frozen chai green tea)

Combine all ingredients in a blender and process well until smooth and creamy.
Serve chilled.

Shopping List

Almond milk
1 cup baby spinach
1 pear

Check the Pantry

Black peppercorns
Cardamom
Cinnamon
Coriander
Ground cloves
Stevia

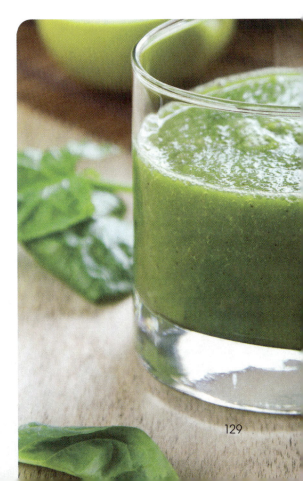

Sunday Brunch

Apple Cinnamon Pancakes   Serves 4–6

The every-once-in-a-while pancakes are a welcome way to start off a weekend. Get a loved one involved, helping you grate the apples or flip the pancakes as you clean up the ingredients from measuring out the batter. These pancakes are a refreshing and rewarding way to start a fall morning with a small crowd!

2 cage-free eggs, well beaten
1½ cups of almond or coconut milk
2 cups gluten-free all-purpose flour
¾ tsp. xanthan gum
1 tsp. baking powder
½ tsp. sea salt
¼ cup coconut sugar
4 medium apples, grated
Zest of 1 lemon
1 tsp. cinnamon
½ tsp. vanilla extract
⅓ cup coconut oil, for cooking
⅓ cup date syrup, maple syrup, or raw honey (optional topping)

Mix eggs with milk in a large bowl.

In a medium bowl sift in flour, xanthan gum, baking powder, sea salt, and sugar.

Combine the wet and the dry ingredients and stir in the grated apples, lemon zest, cinnamon, and vanilla extract.

Heat a thin layer of coconut oil in a large skillet over medium heat. Drop large spoonfuls of batter into the skillet, flattening a bit with the back of the spoon. Cook until golden brown underneath. Flip, press down with spatula, and cook for an additional two minutes or until cooked through.

Serve immediately with syrup of choice. Keep pancakes warm in the oven as you make the full batch!

Photo by Polara Studio

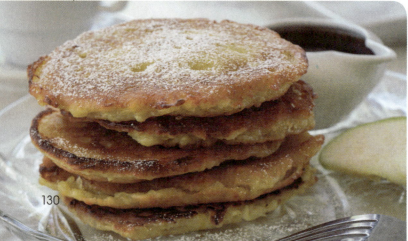

Shopping List

4 medium apples
2 cage-free eggs
1 lemon

Check the Pantry

Almond or coconut milk
Baking powder
Cinnamon
Coconut oil
Coconut sugar
Date syrup, maple syrup or
    honey *(choose your favorite for
    pancakes)*
Gluten-free all-purpose flour
Sea salt
Vanilla extract
Xanthan gum

Sunday Lunch

Asian Chicken Soup   Serves 8

This is a nourishing, soul food soup. I make this at my kitchen often, and enjoy it as a light lunch or dinner anytime I feel like my immune system needs a boost. The richness of chickpea miso (soy free!) adds depth. Add dried astralagus root if you can find it.

¼ cup refined sesame oil
8 slices ginger, peeled
2 yellow onions, sliced
5 chicken thighs or breasts, boneless or meat sliced off the bone
4 cups chopped root vegetables (carrots, turnips, rutabaga, burdock)
½ Tbsp. freshly ground black pepper
1 tsp. salt, to taste
2–3 quarts chicken stock
⅓ cup miso paste
1–2 cups cooked brown rice
    (optional, add in at the end)

Photo by Polara Studio

Spices

½ Tbsp. ginger powder
4 green cardamom pods
1 cinnamon stick
1 piece astralagus root (optional)

Sauté onion and ginger in sesame oil. When slightly browned, add sliced chicken and sauté 5 minutes longer. Add root vegetables and

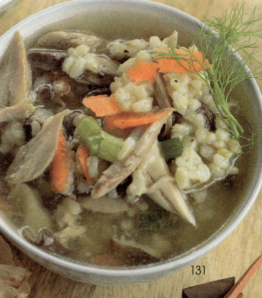

131

spices, then add the stock and bring to a boil. Reduce heat to medium low, and cook for 45 minutes to one hour.

Ten minutes before finishing, stir the miso mixed with a little stock in a small bowl, then add to the soup. Add salt and pepper, to taste. Stir in cooked rice, if desired.

Shopping List

5 chicken thighs or breasts, boneless
4 inches of ginger
4–5 root vegetables
2 yellow onions

Check the Pantry

Astralagus root (optional)
Black peppercorns
1–2 cups cooked brown rice (optional)
Cardamom pods
Chicken stock
Cinnamon stick
Ginger powder
Miso paste
Refined sesame oil (suitable for cooking)
Sea salt

Sunday Dinner

Black Bean Burger With Baked Brown Rice and Shredded Carrot Slaw   Serves 6–8

Black Bean Burger

Forgot to soak the beans? It's OK; you can eliminate this step by using fresh kombu, a seaweed used in traditional Japanese cooking. The kombu deactivates the enzyme inhibitor phytic acid, which causes us to feel bloated if we do not soak beans. Cut a 3-inch-piece of kombu and cover the beans in water, bring to a boil for 5 minutes, then turn off the heat. Drain 2 hours later and proceed to cooking the beans with the kombu.

2 cups black beans, cooked (reserve cooking liquid)
¼ cup extra-virgin olive oil plus more for baking sheet
¾ cup gluten-free all-purpose flour
1 pinch of sea salt
¼ cup chickpea miso
2 Tbsp. coconut oil
1 cup yellow onions, finely chopped
2 cloves garlic, minced
2 tsp. ground cumin
1 tsp. ground turmeric
1 tsp. ground coriander
2 Tbsp. lime juice
¼ cup cilantro, finely chopped
1 tsp. sea salt

Do ahead: Cook the beans, covering them with 1–2 inches of water above bean level. Bring the beans to a boil, skimming off foam with a wooden spoon. Lower heat and simmer for 45 minutes to an hour and a half, until the beans are soft.

Preheat the oven to 350. Lightly grease one baking sheet with olive oil. In a medium bowl, mash the black beans until thick and pasty. Stir in ¼ cup flour, olive oil, a pinch of salt, and the miso. Set aside.

In a skillet, heat coconut oil on medium-high heat. Sauté onions for 5 minutes, stirring frequently. Add garlic and spices. Add lime juice, chopped cilantro, and salt; stir well. Remove from heat.

Add the seasoned and sautéed onions to the mashed beans, adding a few tablespoons of the bean water if needed to achieve a smoother consistency. Stir in remaining ¼–½ cup flour and mix with hands until combined and mixture sticks well together.

Divide the mixture into 6 to 8 burger-size patties. Line burgers on the greased baking sheet and bake for about 20 minutes, flipping once. Serve on gluten-free buns. Freeze extra.

Shopping List

1 bunch cilantro
2 cloves garlic
1 lime
1 yellow onion

Check the Pantry

Brown rice
Chickpea miso
Coconut oil
Dry black beans
Extra-virgin olive oil
Gluten-free all-purpose flour
Ground coriander
Ground cumin
Ground turmeric
Sea salt

Photo by Ben Garvey Photography

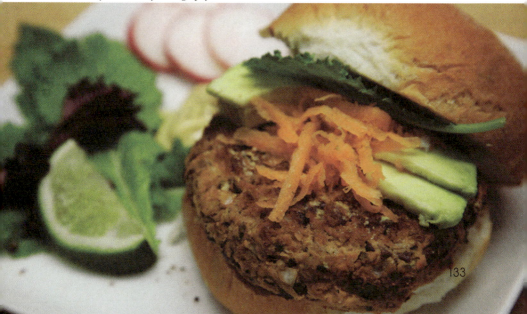

Baked Brown Rice (See Week One: Tuesday Dinner side)

Shredded Carrot Slaw   Serves 4–6

5 large carrots
1 large bulb fennel
½ head green cabbage
¼ cup lemon juice
¼ cup apple cider vinegar
⅓ cup extra-virgin olive oil
Sea salt, to taste
Freshly ground black pepper, to taste
Optional add-ins: ¼ cup chopped parsley, 1 tsp. ground cumin, 2 Tbsp. white
    sesame seeds, 1 Tbsp. raw honey.

Matchstick cut the carrots by hand or with a mandolin (little sticks). Finely chop
the fronds of the fennel bulb. Thinly slice the fennel bulb and cabbage with a
mandolin (or finely chop with a chef's knife). Toss all the vegetables together.

Whisk the dressing ingredients together, taste, and adjust. Toss dressing with
the salad, and season to taste with salt and pepper.

Refrigerate for an hour before serving.

Shopping List	Check the Pantry
½ head cabbage	Apple cider vinegar
5 carrots	Black peppercorns
1 fennel bulb	Extra-virgin olive oil
1 lemon (lemon juice)	Sea salt

Week Three Shopping List

Cooking equipment

- ❏ Bamboo or metal skewers
- ❏ Parchment paper

Cooking wine and vinegar

- ❏ Apple cider vinegar
- ❏ Aged balsamic vinegar
- ❏ Red wine vinegar
- ❏ Rice vinegar
- ❏ Umeboshi vinegar
- ❏ Dry white wine (or more stock)

Dairy and eggs

- ❏ 1 dozen eggs

Dried fruit

- ❏ 3 large dates
- ❏ 1½ cups fresh or dried figs

Dry herbs and spices

- ❏ Black peppercorns
- ❏ Cayenne pepper
- ❏ Ground cloves (optional)
- ❏ Ground cinnamon
- ❏ Cinnamon stick
- ❏ Ground coriander
- ❏ Ground cumin
- ❏ Garam masala
- ❏ Ground nutmeg
- ❏ Dried oregano
- ❏ Crushed pepper flakes (optional)
- ❏ Ground turmeric

Dry or canned pantry items

- ❏ 1 can artichoke hearts
- ❏ Chickpea miso
- ❏ Coconut aminos or tamari
- ❏ 2 cans coconut milk (regular size)
- ❏ Coconut sugar
- ❏ Dulse flakes (optional)
- ❏ Fish sauce (or umeboshi vinegar)
- ❏ Raw honey
- ❏ 1 package kelp (kombu)
- ❏ 1 12-oz. bag kelp noodles (find in refrigerated section of grocery)
- ❏ Maple syrup
- ❏ Molasses

❏ 1 cup pumpkin puree

❏ Red curry paste

❏ Sea salt

❏ Small jar tamarind paste

❏ Umeboshi plum paste

❏ Nutritional yeast

Extracts and sweeteners

❏ Almond extract

❏ Liquid stevia (suggest Sweet Leaf Vanilla Creme)

Fish, poultry, meat

❏ 5 lb. chicken breasts or thighs, boneless and skinless

❏ 1 lb. halibut, deboned and cut into two pieces

❏ 4 6-ounce pieces of salmon (1½ lb.)

Flours

❏ Arrowroot/tapioca flour

❏ Gluten-free all-purpose flour

Fresh herbs and spices

❏ 4 bay leaves

❏ 3 bunches basil

❏ 1 bunch chives

❏ 2 bunches cilantro

❏ 1 bunch dill

❏ 4 inches ginger

❏ 2 bunches mint

❏ 4 bunches parsley

❏ 2 sprigs rosemary

❏ 1 bunch thyme

Grains and beans

❏ 1 can adzuki beans (or ½ cup dry adzuki beans, cooked)

❏ 1 cup dry amaranth

❏ 1 cup brown rice

❏ 3 cups cooked chickpeas

❏ 2 cups quinoa

❏ 2 cups red lentils

❏ 1 can white beans (or ½ cup dry beans, cooked)

❏ ⅓ lb. pound dried white beans

Nuts and seeds

❏ 3 Tbsp. almonds

❏ 4 cups almond milk

❏ ½ cup cashews

❏ ½ cup shredded coconut flakes (unsweetened)

- ❏ ¾ cup coconut milk
- ❏ ¾ cup walnuts

Oils

- ❏ Coconut oil
- ❏ Extra-virgin olive oil
- ❏ Grape seed oil
- ❏ Unrefined sesame oil

Produce

Fruit

- ❏ 3 apples
- ❏ 2 green apples
- ❏ 3 avocados
- ❏ 1 cup blueberries
- ❏ 11 lemons
- ❏ 1 cup lemon juice (or 4–5 more lemons)
- ❏ 6 limes
- ❏ 1 orange
- ❏ 2 pears

Vegetables

- ❏ 4 beets (1 lb.)
- ❏ 1 head bok choy
- ❏ 4 cups braising mix (¼ lb.)
- ❏ 3 lb. broccoli
- ❏ 18 carrots (4 lb.)

- ❏ 2 bunches celery + 3 ribs
- ❏ 7 cucumbers
- ❏ 1 English cucumber
- ❏ 4 heads fennel
- ❏ 3 heads garlic
- ❏ 1 dark green lettuce leaf (you can use a red leaf lettuce; see below)
- ❏ 1 bunch of kale, chard, or collards (your choice)
- ❏ 5 bunches kale
- ❏ 2 lb. parsnips
- ❏ 1 bunch radish
- ❏ 1 head red cabbage
- ❏ 2 heads red leaf lettuce
- ❏ 2 red onions
- ❏ 12 cups mixed salad greens (¾ lb.)
- ❏ 5 bunches scallions
- ❏ 4 shallots
- ❏ 1 large spaghetti squash
- ❏ 1 lb. spinach
- ❏ 4 sweet potatoes
- ❏ 6 cups turnips
- ❏ 2 lb. root vegetable of choice (parsnip, rutabaga, turnip, etc.)

❏ 1 bunch watercress

❏ 5 large yellow onion

❏ 2 zucchini

Stocks

❏ 5 quarts vegetable or chicken stock

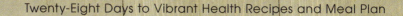

Week Three Menu and Recipes

Monday Breakfast

Waldorf Twist   Serves 1

Granny Smith apples have a slightly higher potassium content than other types of apples. Potassium keeps fluids balanced in and around cells, which is vital to daily electrical flow through your body. If you don't get enough potassium each day, you may wind up having an irregular heartbeat.

1 green apple
3 ribs of organic celery with leaves
1 lemon, peeled if not organic

Cut produce to fit your juicer's feed tube. Juice ingredients and stir. Pour into a glass and drink as soon as possible.

Shopping List

1 green apple
1 bunch of celery
1 lemon

Monday Lunch

Mediterranean Quinoa Salad With Parsnip Fries   Serves 4

Mediterranean Quinoa Salad

1 cup dry quinoa
6 scallions, thinly sliced
2 cups Italian parsley, finely chopped
⅔ cup fresh mint, finely chopped
2 cucumbers, seeded and finely chopped
2 cups baby spinach
½ cup extra-virgin olive oil
½ cup lemon juice
½ tsp. sea salt (or more to taste)
1 tsp. ground cumin
1 cup cooked chickpeas
2 cooked chicken breasts, sliced (optional)

Bring 2 cups of water and quinoa to a boil, uncovered. Place a lid on, lower heat and simmer 15 minutes. Turn off heat and allow quinoa to steam 5 minutes. Remove lid and fluff with a fork.

Meanwhile, chop your salad vegetables and cook your chicken, if opting to use: poach, steam, or roast the chicken.

Combine all quinoa salad ingredients in a bowl and enjoy immediately or keep in the fridge—great chilled for an easy salad in one meal!

Shopping List	Check the Pantry
2 chicken breasts	Chickpeas
2 cucumbers	Ground cumin
1 bunch mint	Extra-virgin olive oil
1 punch parsley	Lemon juice
1 bunch scallions	Quinoa
2 cups spinach	Sea salt

Parsnip Fries

Substitute parsnips in place of carrots in the "Carrot Fries" recipe. (See Week Two: Tuesday lunch side.)

Monday Dinner

Garlic Roasted Shrimp and Broccoli Served With Scallion Quinoa   Serves 4

2 lb. broccoli, cut into small florets
3 cloves garlic, minced
2 lb. wild shrimp, shelled and deveined
2 Tbsp. umeboshi vinegar
2 Tbsp. coconut aminos or tamari
2 Tbsp. tapioca flour
¾ tsp. sea salt
½ tsp. freshly ground black pepper
⅓ cup melted coconut oil
2 cups cooked quinoa
1 bunch scallions, sliced thinly on the bias
Squeeze of lemon (optional)

Preheat oven to 425 degrees.

Toss together broccoli, garlic, 2 tablespoons of the oil, and half the salt and pepper amounts. Spread broccoli out on a baking sheet and roast for 10 minutes.

Meanwhile in a separate bowl toss together remaining oil, salt, pepper, umeboshi vinegar, aminos or tamari, and tapioca flour, stirring until combined evenly. Rinse the shrimp well and toss in this mixture.

Add the shrimp to the baking sheet (or to a new baking sheet if you need more space) and roast for 10 more minutes, tossing once halfway to ensure shrimp cooks evenly.

Season shrimp and broccoli with a squeeze of lemon juice if desired, and serve over warm, cooked quinoa and scallions.

To cook quinoa: Combine 2 cups water with 1 cup dry quinoa and bring to a boil. Cover and simmer on low for 20 minutes. Toss with chopped scallions and serve alongside shrimp and broccoli.

Shopping List	Check the Pantry
2 lb. broccoli	Black peppercorns
1 lemon (optional)	Coconut aminos or tamari
1 bunch scallions	Garlic
1 lb. wild shrimp, peeled and deveined	Grape seed oil
	Quinoa
	Sea salt
	Umeboshi vinegar

Tuesday Breakfast

Cherie's Morning Blend   Serves 2

Celery reduces inflammation. If you are suffering from joint pain, lung infections, asthma, or acne, eating more celery will bring much-needed relief. It also helps you calm down and relieves stress. The minerals in celery, especially magnesium, and its essential oil soothes the nervous system. If you enjoy celery in the evening, you will sleep better.

4–5 carrots, scrubbed well, tops removed, ends trimmed
4 dark green leaves, such as chard, kale, or collards
2 stalks of celery with leaves
1 large cucumber, peeled if not organic
1 lemon peeled, if not organic
1-inch-piece ginger root

Cut produce to fit your juicer's feed tube. Juice ingredients and stir. Pour into a glass and drink as soon as possible.

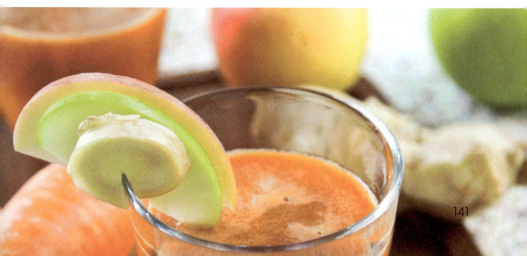

Shopping List

4–5 carrots
2 stalks of celery with leaves
1 large cucumber
1-inch-piece ginger root
4 dark green leaves, such as
    chard, kale, or collards
1 lemon

Tuesday Lunch

Turnip Couscous With Lentil Dahl and a Cucumber Pickle
Serves 4

Turnip Couscous

6 cups turnips, roughly chopped 1-inch cubes
½ cup cashews
1 Tbsp. plus 1 tsp. sea salt
2 Tbsp. rice vinegar

Place the turnips and cashews in a food processor and pulse until chopped to the size of rice granules. Work in batches as needed.

Press "rice" mixture in a strainer over a bowl to release a lot of liquid.

Combine "rice" with salt and vinegar and stir. Spread out in a thin layer on a baking sheet and bake at the oven's lowest setting, 150 degrees or less. Dehydrate if that is an option.

For lowest oven baking: 30–45 minutes (until slightly dry)
For dehydrator (115 degrees): 1½–2 hours

Lentil Dahl

1 large yellow onion, small dice
2 garlic cloves, minced
2-inch-piece of ginger, minced (¼ cup)
3 Tbsp. grape seed oil
1 cup red lentils, rinsed and drained
6 cups water or vegetable stock
2 bay leaves
1 whole cinnamon stick
1 cup cilantro, chopped
¾ cup lemon juice
1½–2 tsp. sea salt
½ lb. spinach

Spices

2 Tbsp. ground turmeric
1 Tbsp. garam masala
¼ tsp. ground cloves (optional)

In a medium pot heat oil over medium-high heat. Add onion, garlic, and ginger and sauté until soft, about 3–5 minutes. Add spices, stirring to distribute evenly.

Add lentils, water or stock, bay leaves, and whole cinnamon stick. Stir and bring to a boil. Reduce heat, cover, and simmer for 20–25 minutes until lentils are tender but not mushy.

Remove the cinnamon stick and bay leaves. Add chopped cilantro, lemon juice and salt. Stir in spinach and adjust season as desired with more lemon juice and salt.

Cucumber Pickle

¼ cup apple cider vinegar
2 cucumbers, deseeded and small chop
¼ tsp. sea salt

Combine all ingredients and season to taste. Add cumin seed and cayenne pepper, if desired for added spice.

Shopping List

1 bunch cilantro
2 garlic cloves
2 cucumbers
2-inch-piece of ginger
½ lb. spinach
6 cups turnips
1 large yellow onion

Check the Pantry

Apple cider vinegar
Bay leaves
Cashews
Garam masala
Grape seed oil
Ground cloves (optional)
Lemon juice
Red lentils
Rice vinegar
Sea salt
Turmeric
Water or vegetable stock
Whole cinnamon stick

Tuesday Dinner

Tuscan White Bean and Kale Soup With Kelp Chips
Serves 6

Tuscan White Bean and Kale Soup

This soup is a version of the classic ribolitta, which traditionally contains tomatoes, pancetta, and cheese. My family loves this vegetarian version, and it's a winter staple in my kitchen.

⅓ pound dried white beans, soaked overnight (or quick soaked)
2 Tbsp. extra-virgin olive oil
1½ cups chopped yellow onion
4 cloves minced garlic
1 cup chopped fennel
1 cup chopped celery
2 tsp. sea salt, or more to taste
¾ tsp. freshly ground black pepper
2 tsp. dried oregano
6 cups chopped kale (2 bunches)
¼ cup chopped fresh basil
4 cups stock, preferably homemade
⅓ cup chickpea miso
3 Tbsp. nutritional yeast

Drain the soaked beans and place them in a large pot with 8 cups of water, and bring to a boil. Lower the heat and simmer uncovered for 40 minutes. Add 1 teaspoon of salt and continue to simmer for about 10 minutes, until the beans are tender. Set the beans aside to cool in their liquid.

Meanwhile, heat the oil in a large stockpot. Add the onions and garlic and cook over medium-low heat for 7–10 minutes, until the onions are translucent. Add the fennel, celery, 2 pinches of salt, the pepper, and oregano. Cook over medium-low heat for 7–10 minutes, until the vegetables are tender. Add kale, and basil and cook over medium-low heat, stirring occasionally, for another 7–10 minutes.

Drain the beans, and reserve the cooking liquid. In the bowl of a food processor fitted with a steel blade, puree half of the beans with a little of their liquid. Add to the stockpot, along with the remaining whole beans. Measure 4 cups bean cooking liquid, and add into the soup along with 4 cups stock. Bring to a boil. Reduce the heat and simmer over low heat for 20 minutes.

Dissolve the miso in a small amount of hot water, then add into the soup along with the nutritional yeast. Taste for seasoning.

Shopping List

2 bunches basil
1 bunch celery
1 head fennel
½ head garlic
2 bunches kale
4 cups stock
⅓ pound dried white beans
1 large yellow onion

Check the Pantry

Black peppercorns
Chickpea miso
Dried oregano
Extra-virgin olive oil
Nutritional yeast
Sea salt

Kelp Chips Serves 4

Kelp is a wondrous source of trace minerals and iodine, like all sea vegetables. It can help protect the body from radiation and supports your adrenal glands. Here is a tasty, crunchy way to get sea vegetables into your weekly diet!

6 6-inch pieces of kelp (also known as kombu)
⅓ cup grape seed or coconut oil

Remove excess salt from kelp with a lightly dampened paper towel by quickly wiping the pieces. Don't get the kelp too wet! Use scissors to cut the kelp pieces in 2-inch by 1-inch pieces. You should have about 20 pieces.

Heat the oil over high heat until very hot. Add the kelp strips to the hot oil, and fry for 3 minutes, flipping once, until the color changes to a deep golden-brown and the kelp curls up and is crispy.

Remove and drain on paper towels. Repeat until all pieces are finished. Enjoy within 1 day for best results! Try with a dipping sauce or alongside a salad.

Shopping List

1 package kelp (kombu)

Check the Pantry

Grape seed or coconut oil

Wednesday Breakfast

Kale Pear Smoothie   Serves 2

Kale is packed with calcium in a form that is assimilated by the body far better than the calcium in dairy products—and that's a great bonus for your bones. Dairy is a pro-inflammatory food for many people, therefore it's important to eat plenty of greens to get your calcium.

1 cucumber, peeled if not organic
1 cup chopped kale
2 pears (Asian or Bartlett)
1 avocado
6 ice cubes

Chop cucumber, kale, and pear and place in the blender and process until smooth. Add the avocado and ice and blend until creamy.

Shopping List

1 avocado
1 cucumber
1 bunch kale
2 pears (Asian or Bartlett)

Wednesday Breakfast

Amaranth Pumpkin Porridge   Serves 4

Amaranth is one of the "super grains" such as quinoa, boasting a full nutrient panel and lots of protein. Here it's paired with pumpkin to make a rich and creamy breakfast porridge. Enjoy!

1 cup dry amaranth
½ tsp. nutmeg
1 tsp. cinnamon
⅓ cup shredded coconut flakes
¼ cup coconut sugar
2 Tbsp. maple syrup
2 Tbsp. coconut oil
¼ tsp. sea salt
1 cup pumpkin puree
2½ cups almond milk
1 cup water (omit if making "cakes," see below)

Preheat oven to 400 degrees.

Bring all ingredients to a simmer over medium heat, stirring to combine (this takes about 10 minutes). Once the mixture comes to a low boil, turn off heat and cover with a tight fitting lid or foil. Place in the oven.

Bake for 45–60 minutes. Use a hot pad to remove pot from the oven, and stir well, as liquid will sit on the top. Serve immediately or cool and reheat in the morning.

We reheat in a glass or ceramic dish in the oven on 425 degrees for 25 minutes, for a hands-off way to enjoy a seasonal hot breakfast.

To make amaranth breakfast "cakes":

Follow this recipe but omit the water and reduce the almond milk to just 2 cups. Cool the mixture completely in the fridge. In the morning pan fry ¼ cup scoops of this mixture in coconut oil over high heat, pressing down to form little "cakes." Brown 2–3 minutes on each side and drizzle with maple syrup. If the cakes fall apart, try adding 1 egg (or 1 tablespoon flaxseed) and ½ cup gluten-free flour. Enjoy!

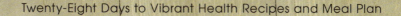

Check the Pantry

Almond milk
Cinnamon
Coconut oil
Coconut sugar
Dry amaranth
Maple syrup
Nutmeg
Pumpkin puree
Sea salt
Shredded coconut flakes

Wednesday Lunch

Kale Fennel and Lemon Salad With Chicken   Serves 4

1 cup radishes, shaved on mandolin or thinly sliced
2 cups fennel, shaved on mandolin or thinly sliced
1 clove garlic, minced
6 cups kale, chopped into bite-size pieces (2 bunches)
Zest from 1 lemon
1 tsp. sea salt
Juice of 1 lemon
1 Tbsp. extra-virgin olive oil
1 lb. chicken breast, cleaned
4 cups water or broth
4 whole black peppercorns
Fennel stalks and fronds (from above fennel)

Combine first 8 ingredients in a large bowl. With clean hands massage the vegetables as if you are squeezing water out of them. Work the vegetables at least 15–20 times until they shrink in size and are well coated. Set aside to rest 20–30 minutes before eating.

In the meantime cook your chicken: bring water or broth to a simmer with peppercorns and fennel. Add a few pinches of salt, and add the chicken to poach for 12–15 minutes, or until cooked through.

Slice chicken and serve overtop the kale salad.

Shopping List

1 lb. chicken breast
2 heads fennel
1 clove garlic
2 bunches kale
1 lemon
1 bunch radish

Check the Pantry

Black peppercorns
Extra-virgin olive oil
Sea salt
Water or broth

Wednesday Dinner

Salmon en Papillote With Lemon and Julienne Vegetables With Roasted Celery Root and Rutabaga   Serves 4

Salmon en Papillote With Lemon and Julienne Vegetables

A great recipe for entertaining! I used to host a family-style dinner for around 45 people every Wednesday night, and I still love entertaining midweek with dinner parties. Make the parchment packets ahead and pop in the oven just before dinner. Be sure packets come to room temperature before cooking, if you do make them ahead (15–20 minutes should suffice).

4 sheets parchment paper
4 6-ounce pieces of salmon or wild cod, pin bones removed
2 Tbsp. extra-virgin olive oil
1 lemon, sliced thinly
½ cup dill
1 medium shallot, julienned (3½ inch length by ¼ inch width, more or less)
1 large carrot, julienned
1 zucchini, julienned
Sea salt, to taste
Freshly ground black pepper, to taste

Photo by Chris Lang

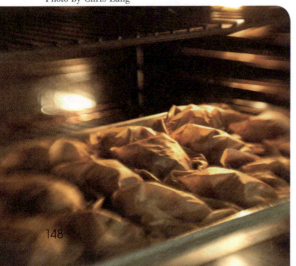

Preheat oven to 425. Cut each parchment sheet into a large heart by folding in half and cutting the exterior of the heart shape using most of parchment sheet. Place open heart shape on cutting board and brush the right side with olive oil.

Place fish onto oiled side of heart, and top with salt, pepper, lemon slices, and herb of choice. Add julienned vegetables on top of herbs, and then drizzle each packet with olive oil and another sprinkle of salt and pepper.

Using a tight rolling technique, fold the packet into a half heart shape, sealing well to ensure steaming will occur. Be sure to fold over the previous fold's edge to create the best results. Repeat with each portion.

Transfer packets to a baking sheet. Bake for 10–12 minutes, until packets puff.

Remove the packets using a metal spatula. Serve directly onto plates and allow guests to open their packets at the table. Fancy and easy!

Shopping List	Check the Pantry
1 large carrot	Black peppercorns
1 bunch dill	Extra-virgin olive oil
1 lemon	Sea salt
Parchment paper (need 4 sheets only)	
4 6-ounce pieces of salmon, pin bones removed	
1 medium shallot	
1 zucchini	

Roasted Celery Root and Rutabaga

1 large celery root (6 inches in diameter)
1 large rutabaga
3 Tbsp. grape seed oil
½ tsp. sea salt

Preheat the oven to 400.

Cut round ends off the celery root so you have a flat, stable surface to peel off the skin. Use a sharp knife to follow the shape of the celery root, peeling downward until all the skin is removed. Chop into 1–2-inch pieces. Chop the rutabaga similarly, though you do not need to peel it.

Place chopped vegetable pieces in a pot and cover with water. Salt the water, turn on high heat, and cover until the water starts to simmer. Simmer for 2 minutes, then strain.

Toss parboiled celery root and rutabaga in a bowl with oil and salt, and then spread out on a baking sheet.

Bake in the oven for 25 minutes or until golden brown. Toss once during cooking time to brown both sides.

Shopping List	Check the Pantry
1 large celery root	Grape seed oil
1 large rutabaga	Sea salt

Thursday Breakfast

Cool Cucumber   Serves 4

Scientists at the University of Ulster revealed that eating watercress daily can significantly reduce DNA damage to blood cells, which is considered to be an important trigger in the development of cancer.

1 handful of watercress
1 dark green lettuce leaf
1 cucumber, peeled if not organic
½ fennel bulb and fonds
1 lemon, peeled if not organic
½ green apple

Cut produce to fit your juicer's feed tube. Wrap watercress in lettuce leaf and push through juicer slowly. Juice all remaining ingredients. Pour into a glass, stir, and drink as soon as possible.

Shopping List

1 cucumber
1 fennel bulb and fonds
1 green apple
1 head dark green lettuce
1 lemon
1 bunch watercress

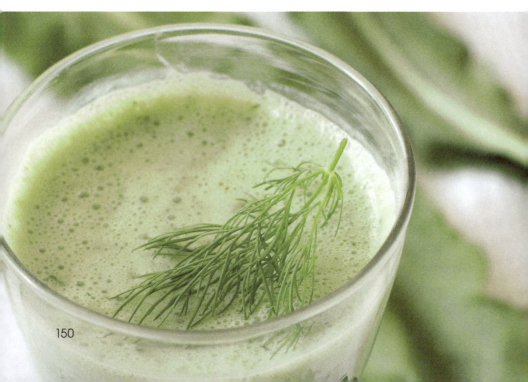

Thursday Lunch

Salmon Salad Wrap With Bright Green Sauce   Serves 4

This is a fabulous summer lunch. Be forewarned—it's messy to eat, but it always hits the spot! During summer when you need to cool the body down but want something a little more than just a plain lettuce salad, this recipe swoops in to save the day. Make the sauce and use for the week on veggies, fish, or on this wrap.

Salmon Salad Wrap

2 Tbsp. extra-virgin olive oil
¼ cup red wine vinegar
1 tsp. raw honey
¼ tsp. sea salt
Freshly ground black pepper, to taste
1¼ pound cooked salmon, chopped
3 stalks celery, finely chopped
1 apple, finely chopped
⅓ cup red onion, chopped
2 heads red lead lettuce
2 carrots, shredded
½ cup bright green sauce (see recipe)

In a small bowl whisk together oil, vinegar, honey, salt, and pepper. Combine salmon and salad ingredients with vinaigrette, and stir to combine well.

Place whole leaves of lettuce on a cutting board and slice leaves lengthwise down the center to make for wraps that are easier to eat. Divide the shredded carrot equally among the leaves in the lower third of the leaf. Next add the salmon salad equally on top of the carrot, about 2–3 tablespoons per wrap. Add one spoonful of bright green sauce over salmon. Carefully roll the lettuce wraps away from you and secure with a toothpick, if packing for later.

Serve with extra bright green sauce on the side. These can be messy but they are so tasty!

Note: Utilize cooked salmon from last night's dinner if there is any left over!

Shopping List

1 apple
2 carrots
3 stalks celery
2 heads red leaf lettuce
1 small red onion
1¼ pound salmon

Check the Pantry

Black peppercorns
Extra-virgin olive oil
Raw honey
Red wine vinegar
Sea salt

Bright Green Sauce   Makes 1 cup

Mix this sauce with brown rice, sautéed vegetables, or drizzle over white fish for a distinctive, tangy flavor. Umeboshi plum paste can be found in the international section of your grocery store or at Asian markets. A little goes a long way—no added salt is needed when you use this amazing paste!

1 bunch scallions, chopped
1 bunch parsley, minced
⅓ cup extra-virgin olive oil
3 Tbsp. umeboshi plum paste
1 Tbsp. chickpea miso, to taste
1 tsp. apple cider vinegar (optional)
1 cup water

Coarsely chop scallions and parsley, and add to blender. Add remaining ingredients and process until smooth.

Shopping List	Check the Pantry
1 bunch scallions	Apple cider vinegar
1 bunch parsley	Chickpea miso
	Extra-virgin olive oil
	Umeboshi plum paste

Thursday Dinner

Tamarind Glazed Chicken Skewers With Brown Rice and Sweet Potato Cakes   Serves 4

Tamarind Glazed Chicken Skewers

Do ahead: Soak bamboo sticks for about 1 hour to prevent them from burning when cooking the chicken. If using metal skewers, coat them in olive oil and set them aside until cooking time.

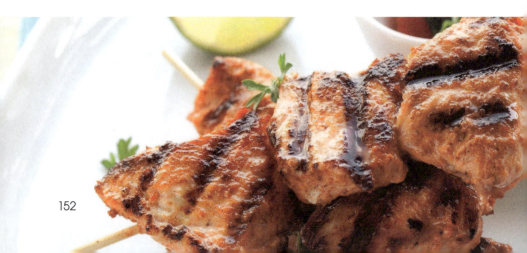

Marinade

1 Tbsp. cumin
½ Tbsp. garam masala
¼ cup extra-virgin olive oil
2 cloves garlic
1½ tsp. sea salt
½ tsp. freshly ground black pepper

Tamarind Glaze

1½ lb. boneless, skinless chicken breast, cleaned, fat trimmed
3 Tbsp. tamarind paste
⅓ cup orange juice
¼ cup molasses
¼ cup honey
¼ tsp. crushed red pepper flakes (optional)
2 Tbsp. lime juice
¼ cup chopped mint
12–15 bamboo or metal skewer sticks
1½ cups fresh or dried figs, halved vertically and stems removed

Make the marinade. Trim the fat off of chicken and cut into 1–2 inch cubes. Toss chicken pieces with the marinade, cover with plastic wrap, and refrigerate overnight. If you are short on time, leave at room temperature for 1–1½ hours and prepare to cook right away.

Make the glaze: In a medium saucepan bring to a boil: tamarind paste, orange juice, molasses, agave or honey, and optional pepper flakes.

Reduce heat and simmer until liquid has reduced to 1 cup, stirring occasionally, about 8 minutes. Remove from heat. Stir in 3 tablespoons lime juice and ¼ cup chopped mint. Set aside.

Make skewers: insert skewers directly into the middle of the chicken and figs. You will fit about 3–4 pieces of chicken per skewer. Brush skewers with ½ of glaze mixture. Discard the marinade.

Bake skewers in the oven on an oiled baking sheet until chicken is cooked through, about 10–12 minutes. Finish with some of the remaining glaze brushed overtop.

Shopping List

1½ lb. boneless, skinless chicken breast
1½ cups fresh or dried figs
2 cloves garlic
1 lime
1 bunch mint
1 orange
Small jar tamarind paste

Check the Pantry

Agave or raw honey
Black peppercorns
Crushed red pepper flakes (optional)
Extra-virgin olive oil
Ground cumin
Ground garam masala
Molasses
Sea salt

Brown Rice and Sweet Potato Cakes

1½ cups cooked mashed sweet potato
2½ cups cooked rice
1½–2 tsp. sea salt
⅔ cup extra-virgin olive oil
½ cup finely diced onion
1 cup gluten-free all-purpose flour (or ⅔ cup brown rice flour and ⅓ tapioca flour)
½ cup coconut oil, for frying

Combine all ingredients and mix well. Test ¼ cup size cake in a pan: coat a small frying pan with an even, light layer of coconut oil over high heat (about ¼ cup to start).

Add cakes (don't overcrowd) and cook for 3 minutes on each side; do not flip until edges are browned around the first side.

Use a metal spatula to flip. Replenish coconut oil as needed. Rewarm in the oven if making ahead.

Alternatively, grease a cookie sheet with coconut oil and bake in the oven on 425, flipping once to brown both sides (about 12 minutes total). Makes 32 cakes.

Note: This recipe freezes well!

Shopping List

1 onion
2 sweet potatoes

Check the Pantry

Brown rice
Coconut oil
Extra-virgin olive oil
Gluten-free all-purpose flour
Sea salt

Friday Breakfast

Coconut Green Delight   Serves 1–2

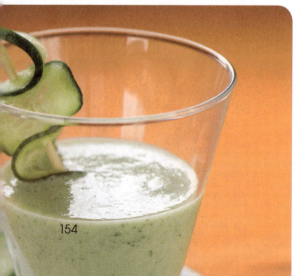

Avocados contain important fats, including phytosterols, which account for a major portion of the avocado's fat. They are key supporters of our inflammatory system and help keep inflammation under control.

1 cup raw spinach
1 avocado
½ English cucumber, peeled if not organic, seeded, and cut in quarters

½–¾ cup coconut milk
Juice of 1 lime
1 Tbsp. powdered greens of choice such as barley greens (optional)
2–3 Tbsp. ground almonds (optional)

Combine all ingredients, except almonds, in a blender until smooth. Sprinkle ground almonds on top, as desired.

Shopping List	Check the Pantry
1 avocado	Almonds (optional)
1 can coconut milk	Powdered greens such as barley
1 English cucumber	greens (optional)
1 lime	
1 bunch spinach	

Friday Lunch

Zesty Lentil Soup With Coriander and Kelp Chips Serves 4

This soup gets its lovely depth from the layering of spices right from the start. Move quickly as you season the oil, which infuses the whole mixture in an intoxicatingly delicious way.

3 Tbsp. coconut oil
1½ tsp. ground cumin
2 tsp. ground coriander
1½ tsp. garam masala
¼ tsp. ground cloves
¾ tsp. sea salt
3 cloves garlic, minced
2 yellow onions, medium dice
½ bunch celery, small dice
5 carrots, small dice
1 cup red lentils
2 bay leaves
8 cups vegetable stock
¼ cup fresh herb of choice (cilantro, basil, rosemary)
¼ tsp. sea salt
1 tsp. ground turmeric
1 Tbsp. red wine vinegar (optional)

Heat coconut oil in a large pot over medium high heat. Add the cooking spices and salt, and stir for 15 seconds. Add the garlic, onion, celery, and

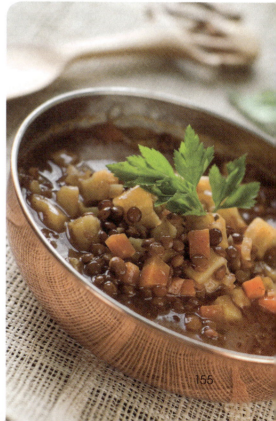

carrots to the pot, and sauté the vegetables for 5–7 minutes or until glistening. Add lentils, bay leaves, and stock. Stir to ensure lentils don't stick to the pot, then bring to a boil. Turn heat to low, partially cover the pot, and simmer for 30 minutes, stirring occasionally.

Stir in salt and turmeric, and taste. Add red wine vinegar if desired, or season with more salt.

Enjoy with Kelp Chips (see Week Three: Tuesday dinner side).

Shopping List	Check the Pantry
2 bay leaves	Coconut oil
5 carrots	Ground cloves
½ bunch celery	Ground coriander
1 head garlic	Ground cumin
Fresh herb of choice (cilantro, basil, rosemary)	Ground garam masala
8 cups vegetable stock	Ground turmeric
2 yellow onions	Red lentils
	Red wine vinegar (optional)
	Sea salt

Friday Dinner

Spaghetti Squash "Pasta" With Lemon White Bean Sauce and Salad With Raw "Caesar" Dressing   Serves 4

Spaghetti Squash "Pasta"

Here is a version of a cream-less "cream" sauce that does not contain nuts or soy. This sauce recipe uses white beans to simulate a creamy consistency along with bright lemon and rich, savory chickpea miso. Roasting the garlic takes this recipe to the next level!

Spaghetti Squash

1 large spaghetti squash (4 lb. or so)
3 Tbsp. grape seed oil
Sea salt, to taste
Freshly ground black pepper, to taste

Preheat oven to 350.

Place whole squash in the oven for 20 minutes to soften the skin.

Once squash is cool enough just to handle, slice lengthwise down the middle and scoop out the seeds.

Rub oil all over squash inside and out, sprinkle with salt and pepper, and place both halves face side down on a baking sheet.

Bake for 30–40 more minutes, until skin is soft to touch and lightly browned.

Once you can handle the squash again, scoop out the flesh from the skin and stir with sauce of choice!

Lemon White Bean Sauce

3 cloves roasted garlic (or 1 raw clove)
¼ cup nutritional yeast
2 heaping Tbsp. chickpea miso
2 Tbsp. extra-virgin olive oil
1½ cups cooked white beans
½ cup water
3 Tbsp. lemon juice (1 lemon)
1 tsp. sea salt

To roast the garlic: cut off the top of the garlic and drizzle with olive oil. Wrap in foil and roast in the oven on 300 for 35 minutes or until softened.

Blend all ingredients together until smooth, and thin with more water if a thinner consistency is desired.

Shopping List	Check the Pantry
1 head garlic	Black peppercorns
1 lemon	Chickpea miso
1 large spaghetti squash	Extra-virgin olive oil
12 oz. can white beans (or ½ cup dry beans, cooked)	Grape seed oil
	Nutritional yeast
	Sea salt

Raw Caesar Dressing

Note: It's important NOT to "cream" the walnuts with the other liquids, as you want them to retain a grainy texture. This is what will give it a cheesy taste. If the dressing needs more "bite" add more lemon juice and sea salt.

¾ cup walnuts, soaked 1 hour
1 Tbsp. extra-virgin olive oil
1½ tsp. sea salt, or more to taste
⅓ cup extra-virgin olive oil
3 dates, pitted and soaked 10 minutes
1 large clove garlic
¼ cup lemon juice (1 large lemon juiced)
1 cup water
1 Tbsp. chickpea miso
2 tsp. dulse flakes (optional)

In a food processor pulse the walnuts, 1 tablespoon oil, and salt until grainy. Do not over blend, you want texture here. Remove from processor and place in small bowl. In a blender combine remaining ingredients and blend until smooth. Remove this mixture and place in the same bowl as the nut mixture. Whisk well until evenly blended. Thin with more water until desired flavor and texture is reached.

For the salad (paired with spaghetti squash): Toss ⅓ cup with 4 heaping cups of greens, and season to taste with more dressing, sea salt, and pepper. Add in various chopped veggies, if desired.

Shopping List

3 large dates
Dulse flakes (optional)
1 clove garlic
4 large handfuls mixed salad
    greens or lettuce
1 large/2 small lemons
¾ cup walnuts

Check the Pantry

Chickpea miso
Extra-virgin olive oil
Sea salt

Saturday Breakfast

Vision Helper   Serves 1

Carrots are rich in carotenes, which are very helpful for strengthening the eyes and improving vision. Blueberries also help improve eyesight, and apples can help remove toxins from the eyes.

3 carrots, scrubbed well, tops removed, ends trimmed
1 cucumber, peeled if not organic
2 kale, chard, or collard leaves
1 cup blueberries, thawed if frozen
½ green apple

Cut produce to fit your juicer's feed tube. Juice the carrots, cucumber, and kale. Turn off the machine and add the blueberries. Top with the plunger. Turn the machine back on and push berries through; then juice the apple. Stir and pour into a glass. Drink as soon as possible.

Shopping List

1 green apple
1 pint blueberries
3 carrots
1 cucumber
1 bunch kale, chard, or collard
    leaves

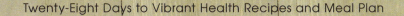

Saturday Brunch

Breakfast Hash With Sweet Potatoes   Serves 4

Use whatever roasted veggies you may have in your fridge to create many variations on this recipe. The template is to combine freshly cooked vegetables with
protein-rich eggs for a power-packed way to start your morning.

2 large sweet potatoes, diced (parcooked and pan roasted first)
3 Tbsp. extra-virgin olive oil
1 small onion, diced (or 1 onion, caramelized)
1–2 carrots or zucchini, diced
2 handfuls spinach or leafy greens, chopped
2 cloves garlic
Pinch of cayenne pepper (optional)
¼ tsp. sea salt plus freshly ground black pepper, to taste
12 eggs
Optional fresh herbs (parsley, oregano, basil, tarragon)

Parcook the potatoes: Place diced sweet potatoes in a pot and add water just to
cover. Add salt and a lid and bring to a boil. Boil for 2–3 minutes and drain. Skip
this step if you already have roasted sweet potato or other roasted veggies you'd
like to use.

Add olive oil to a pan over medium heat. Add all your vegetables and salt and
pepper, to taste. Cook 5–6 minutes, until veggies soften.

Add the eggs and cayenne pepper, and use a wooden spoon to "beat" the
eggs in the pan. Cook 4 minutes, stirring until the eggs are cooked. Add in
optional fresh chopped herbs.

Great served with Dijon mustard!

Shopping List

1–2 carrots or zucchinis
12 eggs
Optional fresh herbs (parsley,
    oregano, basil, tarragon)
2 cloves garlic (optional)
1 small onion
2 handful spinach or leafy
    greens
2 large sweet potatoes

Check the Pantry

Black peppercorns
Cayenne pepper
Extra-virgin olive oil
Sea salt

Saturday Lunch

Warm Salad With Curried Kelp Noodles and Adzuki Beans
Serves 4

Kelp noodles are found in the refrigerated section of most natural health food stores, large and small. They are clear and ready to eat right out of the bag. They have amazing texture and of course, since they are a seaweed, contain lots of important nutrition!

Sauce Ingredients

2 Tbsp. umeboshi plum vinegar
1 cup coconut milk
1 Tbsp. red curry paste
1 Tbsp. coconut sugar
⅓ cup shallots, minced

Salad Ingredients

2 cups adzuki beans, cooked and drained
12 oz. kelp noodles, drained (one bag)
⅓ cup cilantro, chopped
3 scallions, thinly sliced on bias
1 large head bok choy, sliced on bias at ½-inch width

Mix together sauce ingredients and bring to a simmer in a small saucepan.
    Meanwhile place the beans, kelp noodles, chopped vegetables in a large bowl.
    Add heated sauce to coat and season with extra vinegar or curry paste, to your taste. Allow the salad to marinate 10 minutes or more before eating.

Shopping List	Check the Pantry
1 can adzuki beans (or ½ cup dry adzuki beans)	Coconut milk
1 head bok choy	Coconut sugar
1 bunch cilantro	Red curry paste
1 12-oz. bag kelp noodles	Umeboshi plum vinegar
1 bunch scallions	
2 shallots	

Saturday Dinner

Lemon Artichoke Chicken With Crispy Broccoli and Mashed Root Vegetables   Serves 4

2 (whole) boneless, skinless, hormone-free chicken breasts (4 split)
½ tsp. sea salt
½ cup gluten-free all-purpose flour
½ tsp. freshly ground black pepper
2 eggs for 4 chicken breasts
¼ cup extra-virgin olive oil
2 Tbsp. coconut oil
3 Tbsp. white wine
⅓ cup freshly squeezed lemon juice (2 lemons)
½ cup artichoke hearts, chopped (optional)
¼ cup fresh parsley, chopped

Place a chicken breast half between 2 pieces of parchment paper and pound with a meat pounder (flat side) or bottom of a heavy skillet until it is about ¼ inch thick. Repeat with remaining chicken breasts. Sprinkle with ¼ tsp. salt.

Add remaining salt and pepper to flour and mix. Spread the mixture on a large plate. Beat eggs in a bowl. Dip each chicken breast in the egg then the flour to coat on all sides. Place on a plate and prepare remaining pieces.

Heat a large skillet over medium-high heat. Add the olive oil and coconut oil. Once hot place prepared chicken breasts in the pan. Cook for 4 minutes per side or until they are well browned. Transfer chicken breasts to a clean plate and cover until all chicken breasts are browned on both sides and cooked through.

Add the wine and lemon juice to the pan. Scrape the pan to incorporate all the browned bits. Add the artichoke hearts and parsley, and cook until the sauce thickens, about 2 minutes. Pour the sauce over the chicken breasts.

Shopping List

1 small can artichoke hearts
2 (whole) boneless, skinless, hormone-free chicken breasts (4 split)
2 lemons
1 bunch parsley

Check the Pantry

Black peppercorns
Coconut oil
Extra-virgin olive oil
Gluten-free all-purpose flour
Sea salt
White wine

Crispy Broccoli   Serves 4

2 bunches of broccoli, chopped into bite-size pieces
1–2 Tbsp. extra-virgin olive oil
Sea salt
Freshly ground black pepper

Toss all the ingredients together, until well coated. Roast in the oven on 425 degrees until crispy, about 10–12 minutes.

Shopping List

2 bunches broccoli

Check the Pantry

Back peppercorns
Extra-virgin olive oil
Sea salt

Creamy Mashed Root Vegetables   Serves 4

These mashed roots will likely become a favorite in your household for everyday meals as well as holiday celebrations. Surprise yourself with new vegetables! Try celery root (the gnarliest of root vegetables) for a clean, fresh take on this recipe.

2 lb. root veggies (celery root, turnips, parsnips, rutabaga)
2 sprigs of fresh thyme
2 Tbsp. extra-virgin olive oil plus 2 Tbsp. coconut oil
¾ tsp. sea salt, or more to taste
¾ cup coconut milk
1 Tbsp. raw honey (optional)
Freshly ground black pepper, to taste

Peel the vegetables and cut them into medium pieces. Put them in a large (4 quart) saucepan, filling the pan with cold water. Cover the vegetables by 2 inches. Add fresh thyme.

Bring the vegetables to a boil over medium-high heat. Continue to boil until they are easily pierced with a fork, about 25 minutes. Drain and set aside.

In a large bowl toss the vegetables with olive and coconut oil, coconut milk, salt, and optional sweetener. Mash with a potato masher until creamy, adding more coconut milk as needed.

Do ahead option: Keep the mashed veggies warm by holding them in a covered metal bowl set over a pan of simmering water for up to an hour.

Shopping List

1 bunch thyme
2 lb. root vegetable of choice

Check the Pantry

Black peppercorns
Coconut milk
Coconut oil
Extra-virgin olive oil
Raw honey
Sea salt

Sunday Breakfast

Almond Swirl   Serves 2

Peaches contain phenolic compounds that prevent the oxidization of low-density lipoprotein (LDL) cholesterol. It is oxidized cholesterol that is damaging to our bodies. These compounds help fight inflammation associated with metabolic syndrome—a combination of medical disorders that increases the risk of obesity, type 2 diabetes and cardiovascular problems.

1 cup almond milk
2 ripe peaches, pits removed, cut into pieces (if out of season, use frozen peaches)
½ cup kale, chopped
2–3 drops stevia or to taste
1 tsp. pure vanilla extract
½ tsp. pure almond extract
6 ice cubes

Combine all ingredients in a blender and process well until smooth and creamy. Serve chilled.

Shopping List

1 bunch of kale
2 ripe peaches

Check the Pantry

Almond extract
Almond milk
Pure vanilla extract
Stevia (suggest liquid: SweetLeaf
    Vanilla Creme)

Sunday Lunch

Thai Chicken and Apple Salad With Toasted Rice — Serves 4

2 cups apples, cored, thinly sliced, tossed with lemon juice
2 shallots, finely chopped
8 loose cups spinach or salad greens
1 bunch scallions, sliced
1 turnip, thinly sliced
1 cup carrots, matchstick
1 cup torn fresh basil
¼ cup uncooked brown rice (optional)
2 Tbsp. coconut oil
1 lb. chicken breast, sliced
2 Tbsp. gluten-free fish sauce
2 Tbsp. agave nectar or honey
Sea salt, to taste
Freshly ground black pepper, to taste

Dressing

½ cup lime juice
¼ cup coconut palm sugar
3 cloves garlic, minced
1 tsp. sesame oil
2 tsp. fresh ginger, minced

Combine the salad dressing ingredients in a bowl.

Combine the salad ingredients (up to basil) in a large salad bowl. Set aside.

Toast the rice in a dry pan over medium-high until fragrant, about 5 minutes, until it turns a light golden brown and begins to pop. Transfer the rice to a blender or mortar and pestle. Grind the rice down to a coarse powder.

Heat coconut oil in a large pan. Stir-fry the chicken until cooked, about 8 minutes, gradually adding in the fish sauce and agave, 1 tablespoon at time. If the pan becomes too dry, add a little water and cover to steam.

Transfer the chicken to the salad bowl with prepared salad ingredients, heat dressing and toss all ingredients. Garnish with toasted ground rice and torn basil. Salt and pepper to taste.

Photo by Polara Studio

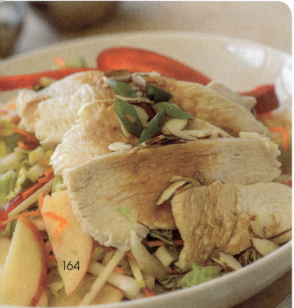

Shopping List

2 apples
1 bunch basil
2 carrots
1 lb. chicken
3 cloves garlic
1-inch ginger
4 limes
1 bunch scallions
2 shallots
8 cups spinach or salad greens
1 turnip

Check the Pantry

Brown rice
Coconut oil
Coconut palm sugar
Gluten-free fish sauce
Raw honey
Pepper
Sea salt
Sesame oil

Sunday Dinner

Halibut and Chickpea Warm Salad With Fresh Herbs and Beet and Caraway Slaw   Serves 4

Halibut and Chickpea Warm Salad With Fresh Herbs

1 lb. halibut, deboned and cut into two pieces
1 tsp. sea salt
Freshly ground black pepper, to taste
3 Tbsp. extra-virgin olive oil
3 Tbsp. red wine vinegar
2 Tbsp. Dijon mustard
¼ cup chopped dill
½ cup chopped chives
4 large handfuls braising mix greens
2 cups cooked chickpeas (or 1 15-oz. can of chickpeas, rinsed well)
1 avocado, sliced

Sprinkle fish with ¼ teaspoon salt and pepper to taste. Place fish in a medium skillet and add water to cover halfway up the side of the fish. Bring water to a boil over medium-high heat. Cover the skillet and cook halibut until opaque and fork tender, about 8 minutes.

Mix olive oil, vinegar, mustard, and dill in a small bowl, and whisk until evenly combined. Toss dressing with remaining salad ingredients in a bowl and season with salt and pepper to taste.

Divide salad between 2 bowls and top with fish. Alternatively, cool fish for 15 minutes in the refrigerator, then enjoy over salad.

Beet and Caraway Slaw   Serves 4

½ head red cabbage, core removed and thinly sliced
4 beets, matchstick cut
1 small apple, matchstick cut (optional)
¼ bunch curly parsley, finely chopped
¼ cup shallot, minced
¼ cup apple cider vinegar
½ tsp. sea salt
1 Tbsp. extra-virgin olive oil (optional)
1 Tbsp. toasted caraway seeds (toast over medium heat in a dry pan until fragrant)

Combine ingredients in a bowl. With clean hands massage the salad firmly, squeezing handfuls at a time. Repeat 20 times altogether. Salad should decrease in size and be coated evenly with the dressing.

Taste and adjust the seasonings to taste. Keep in the fridge for up to 5 days.

Shopping List	Check the Pantry
1 small apple (optional)	Apple cider vinegar
1 avocado, sliced	Black peppercorns
4 beets	Caraway seeds
½ cup chopped chives	Chickpeas
¼ cup chopped dill	Dijon mustard
4 large handfuls braising mix greens	Extra-virgin olive oil
1 lb. halibut, deboned and cut into two pieces	Red wine vinegar
1 bunch parsley	Sea salt
1 head red cabbage	
1 shallot	

Week Four Shopping List

Cooking equipment

- ❏ Bamboo or metal skewers
- ❏ Muffin liners

Cooking wine and vinegar

- ❏ Apple cider vinegar
- ❏ Aged balsamic vinegar
- ❏ Red wine vinegar
- ❏ Rice vinegar
- ❏ Umeboshi vinegar

Dairy and eggs

- ❏ 1 dozen large cage-free eggs

Dried fruit

- ❏ ¼ cup dried currants
- ❏ ½ cup raisins, cranberries, or currants

Dry herbs and spices

- ❏ Black peppercorns
- ❏ Cayenne pepper (optional)
- ❏ Celtic sea salt
- ❏ Curry powder
- ❏ Ground allspice
- ❏ Ground cardamom
- ❏ Ground cinnamon
- ❏ Ground coriander
- ❏ Ground nutmeg

Dry or canned pantry items

- ❏ Almond extract
- ❏ 1 cup almond milk
- ❏ 1 package dried arame seaweed (1 cup)
- ❏ 1 jar artichoke hearts
- ❏ 1 loaf gluten-free bread
- ❏ Gluten-free breadcrumbs (or almond meal)
- ❏ Chickpea miso
- ❏ Coconut aminos or tamari
- ❏ 4 cans coconut milk
- ❏ Coconut sugar
- ❏ Dijon mustard
- ❏ Gluten-free fish sauce
- ❏ Raw honey
- ❏ 1 jar kalamata olives
- ❏ Kelp/kombu
- ❏ Maple syrup
- ❏ Vegenaise or mayonnaise
- ❏ 1 package nori sheets

- ❏ Sea salt
- ❏ Tomatillo salsa (optional)
- ❏ Vanilla extract

Fish, Poultry, Meat

- ❏ 4 lb. boneless, skinless chicken breasts
- ❏ 1½ lb. wild cod
- ❏ ½ lb. smoked salmon
- ❏ 2¾ lb. salmon filet

Flours

- ❏ 1 cup chickpea flour
- ❏ Gluten-free all-purpose flour

Fresh herbs and spices

- ❏ 5 bunches cilantro
- ❏ 2 bunches mint
- ❏ ½ bunch oregano

Grains and beans

- ❏ 3 cups cooked brown rice
- ❏ 2 cups cooked chickpeas
- ❏ 1 cup quinoa

Nuts and seeds

- ❏ 1 cup almonds
- ❏ ½ cup slivered almonds
- ❏ ½ cup cashew pieces

- ❏ 2 Tbsp. flaxseed, ground
- ❏ 1½ cups pecan pieces
- ❏ 1 cup pumpkin seeds
- ❏ ¼ cup sesame seeds
- ❏ ¼ cup black sesame seeds
- ❏ 2½ cups walnuts

Oils

- ❏ Coconut oil
- ❏ Extra-virgin olive oil
- ❏ Grape seed oil
- ❏ Unrefined sesame oil
- ❏ Sunflower oil (for cooking)

Produce:

Fruit

- ❏ 5 apples
- ❏ 6 avocados
- ❏ 1 cup berries of choice
- ❏ 1 cup grapes or banana
- ❏ 9 lemons
- ❏ 4 lime
- ❏ 1 mango
- ❏ 3 pears
- ❏ 2 pippin or other green apples

Vegetables

- ❏ 2 cups arugula
- ❏ ¼ lb baby spinach
- ❏ 1 pint bean sprouts
- ❏ 1 bunch beets
- ❏ 1 head bok coy
- ❏ 3 lb. broccoli
- ❏ 3 inches burdock (optional)
- ❏ 3 lb. butternut squash (whole)
- ❏ 16 carrots (3½ lb)
- ❏ 2 bunches celery
- ❏ 1 bunch collard greens
- ❏ 3 cucumbers
- ❏ 1 head escarole
- ❏ 4 heads garlic
- ❏ 1 green cabbage
- ❏ 3 cups green peas, fresh or frozen
- ❏ 4 cups mixed greens (¼ lb.)
- ❏ 2 Japanese yams (or sweet potato)
- ❏ 2 medium jicamas
- ❏ 2 kale leaves + 1 green lettuce leaf
- ❏ 3 bunches kale + 3 leaves

- ❏ 1–2 kohlrabi leaves or any other dark leafy greens
- ❏ 2 stalks lemongrass
- ❏ 1 bunch mustard greens
- ❏ 1 bunch parsley
- ❏ 2 lb. celery root
- ❏ 1 head radicchio
- ❏ 1 bunch radishes
- ❏ 2 red onions
- ❏ 1 head romaine lettuce
- ❏ 5 bunches scallions
- ❏ 3 cups shiitake mushrooms (¼–½ lb.)
- ❏ ½ lb. spinach
- ❏ 5 turnips
- ❏ 1 bunch watercress
- ❏ 1 yellow onion
- ❏ 3 medium zucchini

Stocks

- ❏ 1 bunch chives
- ❏ 13 inches ginger
- ❏ 1 quart vegetable or chicken stock
- ❏ 1 bunch tarragon

Week Four Menu and Recipes

Monday Breakfast

Pippin Party   Serves 1

The flavonoids in parsley—especially luteolin—have been shown to function as antioxidants that combine with highly reactive oxygen-containing molecules (called oxygen radicals) and help prevent oxygen-based damage to cells. Preventing such damage is very important when it comes to controlling inflammation. We don't tend to eat a lot of parsley, but we can easily juice it.

1 small handful of parsley
1 green lettuce leaf
3–4 carrots, scrubbed well, tops removed, ends trimmed
2 ribs of celery with leaves
2 cloves of garlic
2 pippin apples

Cut produce to fit your juicer's feed tube. Warp parsley in lettuce leaf and push through juicer slowly. Juice all remaining ingredients and stir. Pour into a glass and drink as soon as possible.

Shopping List

2 pippin apples or any green
    apples
3–4 carrots
1 bunch celery
1 head garlic
1 head dark green lettuce
1 bunch parsley

Monday Lunch

Raw Zucchini and Pea Soup With Turnip Noodles   Serves 4

Raw Zucchini and Pea Soup

3 cups coconut milk
1 cup filtered water
3 cups shelled peas, freshly steamed or frozen
3 cups zucchini, chopped
½ cup lemon juice
3 cloves garlic, minced
2 tsp. fresh ginger, minced
3 cups avocado, mashed
½ cup celery, chopped
½ tsp. cayenne pepper
1 Tbsp. sea salt (or more to taste)
3 Tbsp. raw honey
¼ cup mint, destemmed

Turnip Noodles

2 small turnips
Sea salt, to taste

Set aside one cup of peas. Combine all remaining ingredients in a blender and process until smooth. Add up to 2 cups water as desired to thin out the texture.

Pour into serving bowls. Top with remaining peas and optional turnip noodles for garnish.

To make turnip noodles: use a spiralizer or a peeler to make long ribbons of turnip. Season with salt and add to soup for a garnish.

Serve soup chilled or lightly heated.

Shopping List

2 large avocadoes
2 stalks celery
3 cloves garlic
1-inch ginger
3 cups green peas, fresh or
   frozen
½ cup lemon juice
1 bunch mint
2 small turnips
3 medium zucchini

Check the Pantry

Cayenne pepper
Coconut milk
Raw honey
Sea salt

Monday Dinner

Roasted Wild Cod With Olive Vegetable Medley   Serves 4

Roasted Wild Cod

1½ lb. wild cod
2 Tbsp. grape seed oil
¼ tsp. sea salt
Freshly ground black pepper, to taste
1 tsp. dried oregano, optional
1 lemon
3 Tbsp. extra-virgin olive oil
3 cloves garlic, chopped
2 turnips, medium chop
2 heads broccoli, chopped into bite-size florets
½ bunch kale, destemmed and chopped
2 carrots, sliced on the bias
½ cup olive juice

Preheat oven to 425.

Remove pin bones from the cod and cut into four portions. Season fish with a brush of grape seed oil, a sprinkle of salt, pepper, and oregano. Roast in the oven for 12–15 minutes or until cooked through.

Finish with a squeeze of lemon and serve immediately.

Vegetable Medley

Heat the olive oil over medium-low heat in a skillet with a tight-fitting lid. Add the garlic and ¼ tsp. sea salt, 15 seconds.

Add the vegetables and olive juice and shake the pan lightly to divide the liquid evenly on the bottom of the pan. Cover and steam, shaking once or twice.

Steam veggies for 5–7 minutes or until cooked through. Season with more olive juice or salt, as desired.

Shopping List	Check the Pantry
2 heads broccoli	Black peppercorns
2 carrots	Dried oregano
1½ lb. wild cod	Extra-virgin olive oil
3 cloves garlic	Grape seed oil
1 bunch kale	Olive juice (from a jar of olives)
1 lemon	Sea salt
2 turnips	

Tuesday Breakfast

Mean Green   Serves 1–2

Pears contain the phytonutrients that have been shown to provide anti-inflammatory benefits. They have been associated with decreased risk of several common diseases associated with chronic inflammation and excessive oxidative stress.

2–3 kohlrabi leaves
2 ribs of celery
1 cucumber, peeled if not organic
1 pear
½ lemon, peeled if not organic

Place some green leaves in your juicer; alternate leaves with celery followed by cucumber, pear, and lemon. Stir the juice and drink as soon as possible.

Shopping List

1 kohlrabi with leaves (use the
    bulb— chopped up in a
    salad)
1 bunch celery (use remainder
    in other recipes)
1 cucumber
1 pear
1 lemon

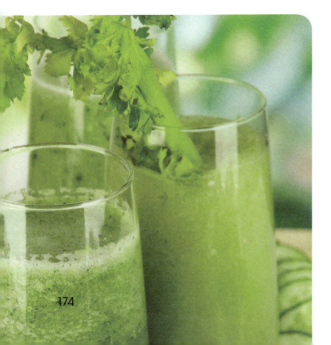

Tuesday Lunch

Mango Mint Quinoa With Spiced Curry Chickpeas   Serves 4

1 lime, zested and juiced
¼ cup fresh cilantro, chopped
½ tsp. sea salt
½ tsp. coarsely ground black pepper
1 cup dry quinoa
1 cucumber, deseeded and diced
1 large handful mint, finely chopped
1 mango, peeled and diced
1 tsp. raw honey
2 Tbsp. coconut oil, melted
2 cups cooked chickpeas (or 1 15-oz. can)
2 Tbsp. extra-virgin olive oil
3 Tbsp. curry powder

Mango Mint Quinoa

Combine the lime zest and juice, cilantro, salt, and pepper in a small bowl.

Cook the quinoa: combine 1 cup dry quinoa with 2 cups water and ½ teaspoon salt. Bring to a boil, reduce heat to a simmer, cover and cook for 15 minutes. Remove from heat and steam 5 minutes more, then remove lid and fluff quinoa with a fork.

While quinoa cooks, chop cucumber, mint, and mango. Season with honey and more salt and pepper, to taste. Combine with cooked quinoa and coconut oil, stirring to combine.

Enjoy with spiced curry chickpeas.

Spiced Curry Chickpeas

Preheat the oven to 300 degrees.

After you have rinsed and drained the chickpeas, leave them to pat dry with a cloth. Mix olive oil, curry powder, salt, and pepper in a large bowl then add the chickpeas and toss to coat evenly. Arrange them in one layer on a lined baking sheet and put it on the lowest rack in the oven.

Bake for 20 minutes, shaking the pan half way through. Cool before enjoying.

Shopping List	Check the Pantry
2 cups cooked chickpeas (or 1 15-oz can)	Black peppercorns
½ bunch cilantro	Coconut oil
1 cucumber	Curry powder
1 lime	Extra-virgin olive oil
1 mango	Raw honey
1 large handful mint	Dry quinoa
	Sea salt

Tuesday Dinner

Mediterranean Chicken and Olives With Wilted Spinach and Escarole Salad   Serves 4–6

Mediterranean Chicken and Olives

¼ cup grape seed oil.
1 small yellow onion, chopped
5 garlic cloves, minced
1¼ lb. boneless, skinless chicken breasts, sliced into 1-inch pieces
1 Tbsp. fresh oregano, destemmed
⅓ cup pitted kalamata olives, coarsely chopped
1 jar artichokes in water, coarsely chopped
2 cups vegetable or chicken stock
2 Tbsp. red wine or red wine vinegar
½ tsp. sea salt
Freshly ground black pepper, to taste
¼ cup fresh basil, destemmed and coarsely chopped

Preheat the oven to 375.

Heat a heavy skillet that can transfer to the oven over medium-high heat. Add the oil, onion, and garlic with a pinch of salt. Cook for 2–3 minutes then add the chicken and cook until it begins to brown, about 4 minutes.

Add the remaining ingredients apart from the fresh basil, stirring to coat the chicken evenly. Cover and transfer to the oven to cook for 20–25 minutes. Remove from oven and stir in chopped basil. Season to taste.

Wilted Spinach and Escarole Salad   Serves 4

2 Tbsp. extra-virgin olive oil
½ lb. spinach
1 head Italian escarole, chopped
1 Tbsp. raw honey
¼ cup dried currants
¼ tsp. sea salt

Heat a medium skillet over medium-low heat, then add the olive oil. Add the spinach and escarole in 2 batches; as the first batch wilts add the second in, when there is room.

When all the greens are bright and lightly wilted, add in the honey, currants, and salt. Sauté for 3–4 minutes, and season to taste. Serve the chicken overtop of the wilted salad.

Shopping List

¼ cup fresh basil, destemmed
and coarsely chopped
1¼ lb. boneless, skinless chicken
breasts, sliced into 1-inch
pieces
1 head Italian escarole, chopped
5 garlic cloves, minced
1 Tbsp. fresh oregano,
destemmed
½ lb. spinach
1 small yellow onion, chopped

Check the Pantry

Artichokes in water
Black peppercorns
Dried currants
Grape seed oil
Pitted kalamata olives
Extra-virgin olive oil
Raw honey
Red wine or red wine vinegar
Sea salt
Vegetable or chicken stock

Wednesday Breakfast

Cranberry-Cucumber Fat Buster   Serves 1

A 2012 study found that cranberry, lingonberry, and blackcurrant juices reduce compounds that promote inflammation.

2 pears, Bartlett or Asian
1 cucumber, peeled if not organic
½ cup loosely packed baby spinach
½ lemon, peeled if not organic
2 Tbsp. cranberries, fresh or frozen
1-inch-piece ginger root
6 ice cubes (optional)

Chop up pears and cucumber and blend until smooth. Add lemon juice, cranberries, ginger, and ice as desired, and blend until creamy.

Shopping List

½ cup baby spinach
1 cucumber
1 lemon
1-inch-piece ginger root
2 pears
1 bag fresh or frozen cranberries

Wednesday Breakfast

Smoked Salmon Frittata Muffins   Serves 4

A delightful weekend breakfast that serves well as a breakfast on the go, for day trips, or as leftovers to start the week off on the right foot!

8 large organic eggs
½ cup coconut milk
2 Tbsp. extra-virgin olive oil, plus more for muffin liners
½ cup red onion, finely chopped
½ lb. smoked salmon, flaked into pieces
8 scallions, thinly sliced
¼ tsp. sea salt
Freshly ground black pepper, to taste

Preheat oven to 325 degrees.
   Beat eggs and coconut milk until evenly mixed.
   In a small pan over medium heat add 1 tablespoon olive oil. Sauté onion for 3 minutes with salt and pepper, to taste. Turn off heat and add the salmon, scallions, and cooked onions to the eggs, stirring to combine.
   Lightly grease 8 muffin tins with remaining 1 tablespoon olive oil (or if using muffin liners, grease the inside of the liners). Evenly divide the egg mixture so it fills ¾ of the way up on each muffin; fill extra muffin tins if there is extra batter.
   Bake for 15 minutes, until puffed and golden brown. Cool and enjoy.

Shopping List

8 large organic eggs
1 small red onion
½ lb. smoked salmon, flaked
   into pieces
1 bunch scallions

Check the Pantry

Black peppercorns
Coconut milk
Extra-virgin olive oil
Muffin liners (if using)
Muffin pan
Sea salt

Wednesday Lunch

Miso Tonic Soup With Brown Rice and Apple-Walnut Charoset   Serves 4

Miso Tonic Soup With Brown Rice

This tonic will help you stay balanced when you feel spacey or on the verge of sickness. Double the recipe so you have leftovers for a couple days.

4 cups vegetable stock
2 cups water
2 2-inch-pieces kelp
1-inch piece of ginger, sliced and smashed lightly
2 stalks lemongrass (use lower ⅓, smash to release flavor)
4 green onions, thinly sliced
2 cups arugula
2 cups cooked brown rice
3 Tbsp. chickpea miso, stirring in a small amount of hot water
2 Tbsp. lemon juice (juice of 1 small lemon)
Sea salt, to taste

Heat stock and water with kelp, ginger, lemongrass, and bring to a boil. Lower heat and simmer 10 minutes. Strain out kelp, ginger, and lemongrass, if desired. Add in green onions and arugula, simmering 2 minutes.

Turn off heat, and stir in miso, lemon juice, and taste. Add in the cooked rice, salt, or more lemon as desired.

Shopping List	Check the Pantry
2 cups arugula	Brown rice
1-inch piece of ginger	Chickpea miso
1 lemon	Kelp
2 stalks lemongrass	Sea salt
1 bunch scallions	Vegetable stock

Apple-Walnut Charoset   Serves 4

3 medium Gala or Fuji apples, peeled, cored, and finely diced
1½ cups walnut halves, lightly toasted, cooled, and coarsely chopped
¼ cup apple cider vinegar
½ cup fresh mint or cilantro, finely chopped
1 Tbsp. raw honey

In large bowl stir together all ingredients. Store covered at room temperature until ready to serve.

Shopping List	Check the Pantry
3 apples	Apple cider vinegar
1 bunch mint or cilantro	Raw honey
1½ cups toasted walnuts	

Wednesday Dinner

Asian Chicken Skewers With Rice Noodle Salad   Serves 4

Do ahead: Soak bamboo sticks for about 1 hour to prevent them from burning when cooking the chicken. If using metal skewers, coat them in olive oil and set them aside until the chicken is ready to be put on them.

Marinade

2 Tbsp. sesame oil
1 Tbsp. gluten-free fish sauce
1 Tbsp. rice vinegar
2 Tbsp. lime juice
½ bunch cilantro, finely chopped
2 Tbsp. raw honey
2 cloves garlic, minced
2-inch piece of ginger, minced
½ tsp. sea salt
¼ tsp. freshly ground black pepper
1¼ lb. boneless, skinless chicken breast, cleaned, each breast cut into 8 slices for skewering

Preheat the oven to 475.

Make the marinade. Trim the fat off of the chicken breasts and slice. Toss chicken with all of the marinade ingredients, cover with plastic wrap and marinate 1½ hours at room temperature or 3 hours in the fridge.

Skewer the meat, then place on baking sheets and broil for 7 minutes, or until cooked through (depending on how thick you sliced your meat).

For the Rice Noodle Salad: follow the recipe from Week Two: Friday Dinner, omitting the shrimp to make a vegetarian side dish.

Shopping List	Check the Pantry
1¼ lb. boneless skinless chicken breast	Black peppercorns
1 bunch cilantro	Gluten-free fish sauce
2 cloves garlic	Raw honey
2-inch-piece of ginger	Rice vinegar
1 lime	Sea salt
	Sesame oil
	Skewers

Thursday Breakfast

Veggie Time Cocktail   Serves 1–2

Several studies have identified carrot's polyacetylenes as phytonutrients that can help inhibit the growth of colon cancer cells.

4 carrots, scrubbed well, tops removed
1 handful of rapini or other dark greens
1 lemon, peeled if not organic
1 garlic clove
2-inch-piece jicama, scrubbed or peeled if not organic
1 handful of watercress

Cut produce to fit your juicer's feed tube. Juice ingredients and stir. Pour into a glass and drink as soon as possible.

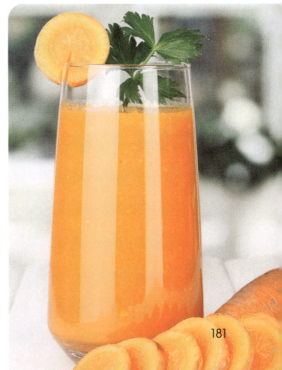

Shopping List

4 carrots
1 garlic clove
1 small jicama (use remainder chopped up in a salad)
1 lemon
1 bunch rapini or other dark greens
1 bunch watercress

181

Thursday Lunch

Scallion Ginger Rice With Spring Kale Vegetable Salad
Serves 4

Scallion Ginger Rice

Soak 1½ cups rice the night before you want to make this recipe. Cook the rice in the morning, and then chill it so you can stir-fry it for dinner. This is the traditional way to ensure your stir-fry rice will not be sticky or creamy.

2 Tbsp. coconut oil
2 cups minced scallions (2 bunches)
3 Tbsp. minced ginger (3–4 inches)
⅓ cup rice vinegar
2 cups bean sprouts
5 cups cooked brown rice, chilled and separated with a fork

Sauce

3 Tbsp. vegetable broth
3 Tbsp. coconut aminos (or tamari)
1½ tsp. pure sesame oil
1½ tsp. sea salt
Freshly ground black pepper, to taste

Mix all sauce ingredients together and set aside.

Heat a large pan or wok over high heat, adding oil until very hot. Add the scallions and ginger and stir-fry 20 seconds. Add the rice vinegar and bean sprouts and toss for 1 minute. Add the rice and stir-fry 2–3 minutes until heated. Add the sauce and toss with 2 utensils to coat the rice and vegetables.

Serve as a side dish, or stir-fry chicken or fish with extra stir-fry sauce (made above) and salt and add into rice for a complete meal.

Shopping List	Check the Pantry
2 cups bean sprouts	Black peppercorns
3–4-inch piece of ginger	Brown rice
2 bunches scallions	Coconut aminos or tamari
	Coconut oil
	Pure sesame oil
	Rice vinegar
	Sea salt
	Vegetable broth

Spring Kale Vegetable Salad   Serves 4–6

This recipe keeps well for 4–5 days in the fridge, so make a big batch and enjoy as a crunchy side dish alongside any meal.

1 bunch radishes, thinly sliced
2 bunches kale, destemmed and chopped into bite-size pieces
2 cups snap peas
1 bunch beets with greens, beets shredded and greens chopped
2 scallions, thinly sliced
2-inch-piece of ginger, minced
¼ cup sesame seeds
3 Tbsp. lemon juice
2 Tbsp. extra-virgin olive oil
½ tsp. sea salt

Combine all ingredients in a large bowl. With clean hands massage the vegetables as if you are squeezing water out of them. Work the vegetables at least 15 times.

After 10 minutes work the vegetables another 15 times and taste. Finish the recipe at this point, or repeat the process 1 more time.

Shopping List

1 bunch beets
2-inch-piece of ginger
2 bunch kale
1 bunch radishes
½ bunch scallions
2 cups snap peas

Check the Pantry

Lemon juice (or 2 lemons)
Extra-virgin olive oil
Sea salt
Sesame seeds

Thursday Dinner

Maple Pecan Crusted Salmon With Mashed Celery Root and Steamed Broccoli Rabe   Serves 4

Drum roll, please. This is a favorite recipe of customers and family alike! A friend of my mother's, who was a former professional chef and a dancer (like me), created the original recipe. I've adapted it slightly, and this recipe is still big crowd pleaser. I hope you will enjoy it as we do, for family dinners as well as for special occasions.

Maple Pecan Crusted Salmon

1½ lb. salmon filet, deboned
Extra-virgin olive oil for brushing fish
¼ tsp. sea salt
Freshly ground black pepper, to taste

Topping

¼ cup maple syrup
1 cup pecan pieces
1 tsp. freshly ground black pepper
½ tsp. sea salt

Preheat the oven to 325.

In a food processor pulse topping ingredients until fine and evenly textured. Place the salmon on a lined baking sheet. Brush the salmon with olive oil and season with salt and pepper. Press the maple pecan topping evenly over the salmon filet. Bake the salmon filet for 25–30 minutes, or until cooked through in the center.

Portion out into 4 servings or serve whole as an appetizer with Belgian endive.

Shopping List

1½ lb. salmon filet, deboned

Check the Pantry

Black peppercorns
Extra-virgin olive oil
Maple syrup
Pecan pieces
Sea salt

Mashed Celery Root   Serves 4

2 lb. celery root
2 Tbsp. extra-virgin olive oil
2 Tbsp. coconut oil
1 cup coconut milk
¾ tsp. sea salt (or more to taste)
Freshly ground black pepper, to taste

Peel the vegetables and cut them into medium pieces. Put them in a large (4 quart) saucepan, filling the pan with cold water. Cover the vegetables by 2 inches.

Bring the vegetables to a boil, covered, over high heat. Continue to boil until they are easily pierced with a fork, about 15–20 minutes. Drain and place in a large bowl. Add the oils, coconut milk, salt, and pepper. Mash with a potato masher until creamy, adding more salt if desired.

Do ahead option: Keep the mashed veggies warm by keeping them in a covered metal bowl set over a pan of simmering water for up to 1 hour (double boiler).

Steamed Broccoli Rabe   Serves 4

2 lb. broccoli, cut into small florets
½ tsp. sea salt, for boiling water

Boil 2 inches of water in a pot, and add ¼ teaspoon salt and the broccoli florets (in a steaming basket or just add to the water).

Cover with a tight-fitting lid and steam for 3–4 minutes. Drain and enjoy immediately, or cool under cold running water if enjoying later.

Shopping List	Check the Pantry
2 lb. broccoli 2 lb. celery root	Black peppercorns Coconut milk Coconut Oil Extra-virgin olive oil Sea salt

Friday Breakfast

Sprouted Almond-Vanilla Smoothie   Serves 1–2

One-quarter cup of almonds contains almost 99 mg of magnesium. Studies show that a deficiency of magnesium is associated with heart attack, and that immediately following a heart attack, lack of sufficient magnesium promotes free-radical injury to the heart.

1 cup raw almonds, soaked overnight
1 cup almond milk
1 cup berries (blueberries, raspberries, or blackberries)
½ tsp. pure vanilla extract
6 ice cubes

Soak almonds in water overnight so that they will sprout. (Sprouting allows the almond to partially germinate, which removes the enzyme inhibitors and increases nutrient value.) Blend together almonds, almond milk, berries, vanilla, and ice. Pour in glasses and serve as soon as possible.

Shopping List	Check the Pantry
1 cup raw almonds	Almond milk
1 pint berries of choice	Pure vanilla extract

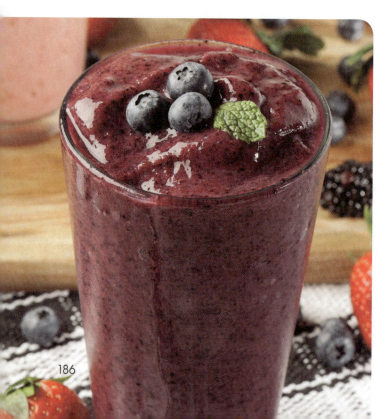

Friday Lunch

Chicken Curry Salad Served in Lettuce Cups With Apple-Walnut Charoset   Serves 4

A delicious salad for lunch or dinner. Recipe by Cherie!

½ cup Veganaise or mayonnaise
1 tsp. fresh lemon juice
2 Tbsp. curry powder
2 cups cooked chicken, chopped
¼ cup diced celery
½ cup chopped cilantro
¼ cup slivered almonds
1 head romaine lettuce or green leaf lettuce

Blend mayonnaise, lemon juice, and curry powder. Put the remaining ingredients (except lettuce) into a medium to large salad bowl and toss with the Veganaise or mayonnaise mixture. Chill at least one hour before serving.

Serve the chicken salad in the lettuce leaves or tear and toss into the salad mixture.

Note: Walnuts may be substituted for almonds. Also, to enjoy with Apple-Walnut Charoset (see recipe from Week Four: Wednesday lunch).

Shop List	Check the Pantry
½ bunch celery	Curry powder
2 chicken breasts (cooked)	Slivered almonds
1 bunch cilantro	Veganaise or mayonnaise
1 lemon	
1 head romaine lettuce	

Friday Dinner

Wild Salmon Burgers With Cardamom, Avocado, and Radicchio Salad   Serves 4

Wild Salmon Burgers

1¼ lb. salmon, skin removed and chopped
2 cloves garlic
½-inch-piece of ginger
2 Tbsp. Dijon mustard
¼ cup tarragon, chopped
2 green onions, finely chopped
2 Tbsp. chickpea miso, dissolved in 1 Tbsp. warm water
1 egg, beaten
½ cup gluten-free breadcrumbs or almond meal
1 Tbsp. flaxseed, ground
Sunflower oil, for cooking
Sea sat, to taste

Place garlic and ginger in a food processor and pulse until finely chopped. Add the salmon and pulse until evenly chopped. Remove mixture from processor and place in a medium-size bowl.

Add remaining ingredients and gently mix by hand until ingredients are evenly distributed. Form into ¼ cup size balls, flatten into patties, and chill for at least 1 hour or up to 1 day.

Cook on the grill or in a skillet: lightly oil with sunflower oil. Place the patties in the pan (or on grill), do not overcrowd. Cook on medium-high heat for 5 minutes on the first side, then flip and cook an additional 4–5 minutes.

Transfer to a plate, sprinkle with salt, and repeat until all patties are cooked.

Enjoy on a gluten-free bun or on its own with lettuce and a condiment of choice. (I love Dijon mustard!)

Shopping List

½ cup gluten-free breadcrumbs
    or almond meal
1 egg
2 cloves garlic
½ inch ginger
½ bunch green onions
1¼ lb. salmon
1 bunch tarragon

Check the Pantry

Chickpea miso
Dijon mustard
Flaxseed
Sea salt
Sunflower oil

Cardamom, Avocado, and Radicchio Salad   Serves 6

Here is one of my favorite salads to make in cold weather. By heating the salad dressing lightly, you achieve a warming (not cold) salad for winter. Cardamom is the "queen of spices," as it is a favorite spice among women, historically.

Dressing

6 Tbsp. warmed coconut oil
2 cloves of garlic, minced
1-inch-piece of ginger, minced
2 tsp. ground cardamom
1 tsp. ground coriander
1 tsp. umeboshi vinegar
2 tsp. Dijon mustard
1 tsp. raw honey
Sea salt, to taste
Freshly ground black pepper, to taste

Salad

3 stalks celery, thinly sliced on the bias
2 large avocadoes, chopped into 2-inch pieces
6 cups arugula
1 head radicchio, chopped
½ cup walnuts, toasted
Sea salt, to taste
Freshly ground black pepper, to taste

Heat coconut oil over low-medium heat. Add garlic and ginger, stirring for 15 seconds. Add spices and stir 15 more seconds. Add remaining ingredients and stir until just combined and lightly heated.

Toss in a bowl with all salad ingredients until slightly wilted and well coated.

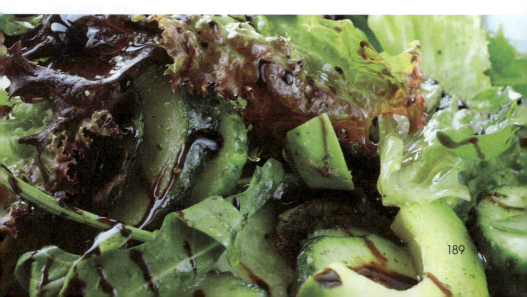

The avocado will make the salad slightly creamy. Season with sea salt and pepper, and serve immediately.

Note: If you are making this dressing to enjoy at a later time, use olive oil as it will not solidify like coconut oil. If you cannot find umeboshi vinegar at your local store (look in the Asian section) then substitute one tablespoon balsamic vinegar.

Shopping List	Check the Pantry
6 cups arugula	Black peppercorns
2 avocadoes	Coconut oil (or extra-virgin olive oil)
3 stalks celery	Dijon mustard
2 cloves of garlic	Ground cardamom
1-inch-piece of ginger	Ground coriander
1 head radicchio	Raw honey
	Sea salt
	Umeboshi vinegar
	Walnuts

Saturday Breakfast

Yucatecan Apple   Serves 1

There is evidence that some inflammatory aspects of obesity may be altered by sulfur-containing compounds in garlic.

2 apples
3 kale leaves
1 garlic clove (no need to peel)
Pinch of Celtic sea salt
Pinch of freshly ground black pepper
Pinch of allspice

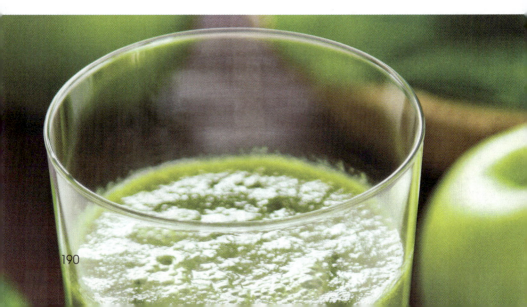

Cut produce to fit your juicer's feed tube. Juice apples, kale, and garlic; stir in spices. Pour into a glass and drink as soon as possible.

Shopping List	Check the Pantry
2 apples	Allspice
1 bunch kale	Black peppercorns
1 clove garlic	Celtic sea salt

Saturday Lunch

Southwest Chicken Collard Wrap With Mexican Cabbage Slaw   Serves 4

Southwest Chicken Collard Wrap

1 lb. boneless, skinless chicken breasts (2)
8 large collard green leaves, middle stem removed
1 cup carrot, shredded
1 cup cucumber, thinly sliced
1 cup cilantro, chopped
2 avocadoes, sliced
Cayenne pepper, to taste
Lime juice, to taste
Sea salt, to taste
Freshly ground black pepper, to taste
1 cup tomatillo salsa (optional)

Poach or roast chicken breasts, as desired, for 12–15 minutes until cooked through.

Slice chicken and season with salt, pepper, cayenne pepper, and lime juice, to taste. Let rest while you prepare your collard wraps ingredients.

Remove middle stem from collard leaves and cut the leaves into 2 pieces lengthwise so you have 4 half leaves per person.

Line up all 16 halves and divide all ingredients between the leaves. Line up a bit of each vegetable ingredient in the lower third of the collard leaf. Add sliced chicken.

Get ready to roll: Fold up the lower end of the collard leaf over the ingredients, and roll the leaf away from you. Secure with a toothpick and repeat on all remaining leaves.

Enjoy with salsa or hot sauce, as desired.

Shopping List

2 avocadoes
2 carrots
1 lb. boneless skinless chicken
     breast
1 small bunch cilantro
1 large bunch collard greens
1 small cucumber
1 cup tomatillo salsa (optional)

Check the Pantry

Black peppercorns
Cayenne pepper
Lime juice
Sea salt

Mexican Cabbage Slaw   Serves 4–6

1 head green cabbage, core removed, thinly sliced
3 carrots, matchstick cut
1 bunch cilantro, minced
1 bunch of scallions, thinly sliced
2 cloves of garlic, minced
⅓ cup lime juice
½ tsp. sea salt
1 Tbsp. extra-virgin olive oil
Freshly ground black pepper or cayenne pepper, to taste (optional)

Combine ingredients in a bowl. With clean hands massage the salad firmly, squeezing handfuls at a time. Repeat 20 times altogether. Salad should decrease in size and be coated evenly with the dressing. Taste and adjust the seasonings as needed.

   Keep in the fridge for up to 5 days.

Shopping List

1 head green cabbage
3 carrots
1 bunch cilantro
2 garlic cloves
Lime juice
1 bunch scallions

Check the Pantry

Black peppercorns
Cayenne pepper
Extra-virgin olive oil
Sea salt

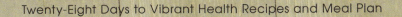

Saturday Dinner

Chickpea Crepes With Arame-Carrot Filling and a Simple Salad With Pumpkin Seeds   Serves 4–6

This is another recipe adapted from my cooking school and chef Myra Kornfeld. I love how easy the crepes are to make, and the filling is packed with amazing arame, my favorite sea vegetable. Go out on a limb and make this interesting recipe. I think you will be pleased with the efforts! Freeze any extra crepe batter.

1 cup chickpea flour
1 cup gluten-free all-purpose flour
1 tsp. sea salt
2 Tbsp. extra-virgin olive oil or coconut oil
2 cups warm water
¼ cup finely chopped chives
½ cup arame, dried
1 red onion, thinly sliced
1 large carrot, shredded
1 tsp. sesame oil
1 Tbsp. chopped ginger
Umeboshi plum vinegar (optional)
Sea salt, to taste
Freshly ground black pepper, to taste

Sift flours and whisk together with salt in a bowl. Add oil and water and whisk to combine until evenly blended. Stir in chives and let batter rest 30 minutes at room temperature. Soak arame for 10 minutes, then drain off water.

In a pan add arame, onion, carrot, sesame oil, ginger, salt, pepper, and a dash of umeboshi vinegar. Add water to almost cover (¾ of the way over ingredients). Bring to a boil, lower heat, and simmer until liquid evaporates, 30 minutes or so.

Photo by Polara Studio

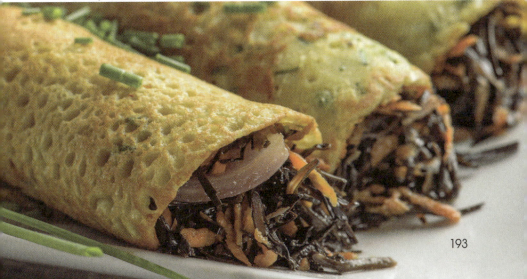

Meanwhile make the crepes: heat a small crepe pan or nonstick skillet over medium heat. Brush pan lightly with oil. Pour a scant ¼ cup batter into pan, swirling to coat bottom evenly. Cook until surface bubbles, 1 minute. Loosen edges and flip. Cook second side for 30 seconds.

To plate, fill each crepe with ¼ cup arame filling and roll. Garnish with chives.

For the Simple Salad With Pumpkin Seeds: Combine ¼ cup olive oil and ¼ cup apple cider vinegar, and add a pinch of salt (and optional cayenne pepper). Add 4–6 handfuls of arugula or mixed lettuce greens, tossing to coat evenly. Season to taste and top with ½ cup toasted, salted pumpkin seeds.

Shopping List

1 bag dried arame
4–6 handfuls arugula or mixed
  lettuce greens
1 large carrot
1 cup chickpea flour
1 bunch chives
1-inch ginger
Umeboshi plum vinegar
  (optional)
1 red onion

Check the Pantry

Apple cider vinegar
Black peppercorns
Coconut oil
Extra-virgin olive oil
Gluten-free all-purpose flour
Sea salt
Sesame oil

Sunday Breakfast

Peppy Parsley   Serves 1

Lemon helps remove uric acid in your joints, which is one of the main causes of joint inflammation.

½ bunch parsley
2 ribs celery
1–2 carrots, scrubbed well, tops removed, ends trimmed
½ cucumber, peeled if not organic
½ lemon, peeled

Cut all produce to fit the juicer and push through the juicer. Drink as soon as possible.

Shopping List

1–2 carrots
1 bunch celery
1 cucumber
1 lemon
1 bunch parsley

Sunday Brunch

Holiday Baked French Toast   Serves 6

Here is a festive weekend breakfast dish perfect for entertaining. Set it up the night before so the bread soaks in all the spices and flavors. Delicious and celebratory, while being naturally gluten and dairy free!

1–2 Tbsp. coconut oil, for greasing pan, and more for topping
1 loaf gluten-free bread (cut into about 1½-inch slices)
½ cup pecans
½ cup raisins, cranberries, or currants
3 cups coconut milk
3 eggs
2 Tbsp. coconut sugar
Zest of 1 lemon
½ tsp. sea salt
1 Tbsp. almond extract
1 tsp. cinnamon
⅛ tsp. nutmeg
½ cup maple syrup, for topping
1 cup sliced fresh grapes or sliced bananas

Oil a 9-by-13-inch baking dish with coconut oil.

In the pan arrange the slices of bread in 2 or 3 tightly packed layers, sprinkling the nuts and dried fruit in between each layer.

Whisk coconut milk, eggs, coconut sugar, lemon zest, sea salt, and almond extract in a bowl. Pour over the bread. Sprinkle with 1 teaspoon cinnamon and ⅛ teaspoon nutmeg.

Wrap tightly with plastic wrap and refrigerate overnight (or at least a few hours).

Photo by Polara Studio

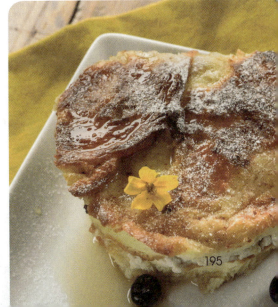

195

Uncover and bake at 400 for 35–40 minutes, or until golden.
Cut into squares and top with maple syrup and fresh fruit.

Shopping List

1 loaf gluten-free bread (cut
    into about 1½-inch slices)
3 eggs
1 cup sliced fresh grapes or
    sliced bananas
1 lemon
½ cup pecans
½ cup raisins, cranberries, or
    currants

Check the Pantry

Almond extract
Cinnamon
Coconut milk
Coconut oil
Coconut sugar
Maple syrup
Nutmeg
Sea salt

Sunday Lunch

All-Vegetable Sushi With Butternut Squash and Spring Kale Vegetable Salad   Serves 8

Holidays are big in my family. I am the youngest of three girls, and to this day we begin planning our menus well in advance, with gusto and a healthy dose of humor too. We also love costuming! I created this version of raw vegan sushi for a fun fall harvest party. Try this recipe for your next get together—costumed or not!

3 cups jicama, roughly chopped into 1-inch cubes
3 cups turnip, roughly chopped into 1-inch cubes
½ cup raw cashew pieces
1 Tbsp. plus 1 tsp. sea salt
2 Tbsp. rice vinegar
1½ cups cooked, peeled, and sliced butternut squash
1 bunch scallions

Photo by Polara Studio

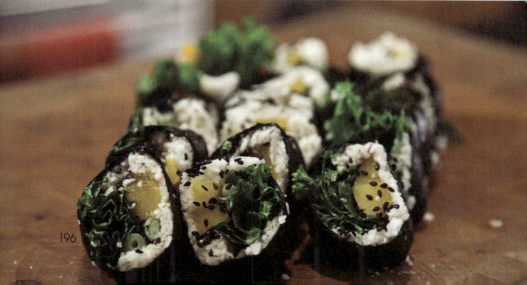

1 bunch mustard greens, destemmed
Black sesame seeds
1 package nori sheets (seaweed)

Place the chopped jicama, turnip, and cashews in a food processor with 1 tablespoon salt, and pulse until chopped to the size of rice granules. Work in batches as needed.

Press "rice" mixture in a strainer over a bowl to release excess moisture. Combine "rice" with remaining 1 tsp. salt and vinegar and stir in strainer to further release moisture.

Lay nori sheets rough side up. Spoon an even layer of "rice" in the lower third of the sheet. Arrange "rice" in a square shape all the way to ¼ inch from the sides.

Line up small amounts of each ingredient in a horizontal line (1 scallion, ½ mustard green leaf, long pieces of cut squash, a sprinkle of black sesame seeds). Roll tightly away from you. Set seam side down and repeat. Slice with a bread knife (serrated) and serve. Wipe knife clean between cuts for better results.

Enjoy with Spring Kale Vegetable Salad (Week Four: Thursday Lunch)

Shopping List

3 lb. butternut squash
1 large jicama
1 bunch mustard greens
1 package nori sheets
1 bunch scallions
½ cup black sesame seeds
2 large turnips

Check the Pantry

Raw cashew pieces
Rice vinegar
Sea salt

Sunday Dinner

Shiitake Mushroom Stir-Fry With Roasted Japanese Yams and Miso Tonic Soup   Serves 4

Shiitake Mushroom Stir-Fry

¼ cup. coconut oil
4 cloves garlic, sliced in coins
3 cups shiitake mushrooms (leave whole if small, slice in half if large)
1 large head bok choy (or 6 baby bok choy heads), sliced on the bias
3 inches burdock, sliced thinly (optional)
1 Tbsp. balsamic vinegar
½ tsp. sea salt
½ cup toasted walnuts or almonds, pulsed until coarse
Freshly ground black pepper, to taste

Mis en place (that is, set up in your kitchen working area) all ingredients, this recipe finishes quickly.

Heat the coconut oil in a wok or skillet until very hot. Add the garlic and brown, 30 seconds. Add the shiitakes, cook for 3–5 minutes until nicely browned. Add the bok choy, burdock, vinegar, and salt. Cook for another 3 minutes. Add the walnuts or almonds, stirring to combine.

Taste and season with pepper and more salt or vinegar, as desired.

Roasted Japanese Yams   Serves 4

Japanese yams have a purple hued skin and a near-white flesh. They are supremely sweet on their own and need very little fussing to make them delicious!

2 large Japanese yams
3 Tbsp. grape seed oil
½ tsp. sea salt

Preheat the oven to 400.

Cut the yams into 1-inch cubes. Toss yams in a bowl with oil and salt, and then spread out on a baking sheet.

Bake in the oven for 35–40 minutes, or until golden brown. Toss once during cook time to brown both sides.

Enjoy with Miso Tonic Soup (Week Four: Wednesday Lunch)

Shopping List

1 large head bok choy (or 6 baby bok choy heads)
3 inches burdock (optional)
2 large Japanese yams
4 cloves garlic
3 cups shiitake mushrooms

Check the Pantry

Balsamic vinegar
Black peppercorns
Coconut oil
Grape seed oil
Sea salt
Walnuts or almonds

Dealer's Choice

Try your favorite dinner recipe from any of the previous weeks! Practice makes perfect, so have a second go at a dinner you loved!

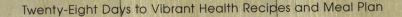
Snacks

Onion Rings   Serves 6–8

4–5 sweet onions (yellow, white, Walla Walla sweets)
¼ cup apple cider or coconut vinegar
¼ cup fresh lemon juice
¼ cup extra-virgin olive oil
2 Tbsp. nutritional yeast
Pinch of sea salt

Cut onions into thin slices and set aside. In a blender add the lemon juice, vinegar, olive oil, and a pinch of salt and process until well combined. Pour marinade over the onions and marinate for several hours. Before placing the onion rings on dehydrator sheets, shake off excess marinade so that the onion rings are not dripping. Sprinkle them with nutritional yeast. Dehydrate at 105–115F for 7–8 hours or until crisp.

Shopping List

1 lemon
4–5 sweet onions

Check the Pantry

Apple cider or coconut vinegar
Nutritional yeast
Extra-virgin olive oil
Sea salt

Dehydrated Zucchini Chips

2 zucchinis
Sea salt, to taste

Slice zucchinis into thin rounds and sprinkle with a little sea salt, as desired. You can also sprinkle them with your favorite seasoning. Place zucchini slices on dehydrator sheets and dehydrate for 7–8 hours at 105 to 115 F or until crispy. They are surprisingly sweet and delicious.

Shopping List

2 zucchinis

Check the Pantry

Sea salt

Dehydrated Tomatoes and Basil

3–4 tomatoes
12–16 basil leaves

Slice tomatoes thinly and put a fresh basil leaf on top of each slice, once you've place them on a dehydrator sheet. Dehydrate for about 12 hours at 105 to 115 F or until crispy.

Shopping List

3–4 tomatoes
1 package fresh basil

Bright Beet Dip   Yields 3 cups

Here is a brilliantly colored and nutritious version of a hummus for dipping raw veggies. It's also great with crackers. A welcome addition to a traditional crudité platter. This is a recipe I've adapted from my mother, who raised me on beautiful home-cooked meals and fresh salads every day.

2 medium red beets, cooked until tender (1½ cups)
1 cup cooked chickpeas
2 cloves garlic
¼ cup almond flour (or slivered almonds, ground)
½ cup extra-virgin olive oil
⅓ cup red wine vinegar
½ tsp. sea salt

Blend all ingredients together in a food processor or blender, adding a tiny bit of water as needed to thin.

Enjoy with raw veggies or on a slice of gluten-free toast, with a quinoa salad or cooked chicken.

Shopping List

2 medium red beets
2 cloves garlic

Check the Pantry

Almond flour or slivered almonds
Chickpeas
Extra-virgin olive oil
Red wine vinegar
Sea salt

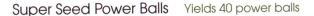

Super Seed Power Balls   Yields 40 power balls

This recipe yields a lot, so you can freeze the balls and grab 4 or so when you need a snack for the day. It's worthwhile to roll them all at once and freeze them or keep them in the fridge (for up to 10 days)

16 oz. pumpkin seed or sunflower seed butter (1 pound)
14 oz. raw honey (just under 2 cups)
3 cups rolled oats
2 cups white sesame seeds (or shredded unsweetened coconut flakes)

Mix the pumpkin seed or sunflower seed butter and raw honey together in a bowl.

Measure oats as they are or blend them until they assume a powderlike texture.

Add the oats to the seed butter/honey mixture and mix until combined, working with hands. Adjust consistency if necessary.

Roll batter into small balls. Wet hands often to prevent mixture from sticking. Roll balls into your choice of sesame seeds or coconut. *Chill and eat!*

Shopping List

1 lb. pumpkin seed or sunflower seed butter

Check the Pantry

Raw honey
Rolled oats
White sesame seeds (or shredded coconut flakes)

Desserts

Raw Vegan "Cheesecake"   Serves 6–8

3 cups raw cashews
½ cup fresh lemon juice
¼ cup coconut nectar or pure maple syrup or 1 Tbsp. coconut nectar with ¼ tsp. liquid stevia
½ cup coconut oil, melted
2 tsp. pure vanilla extract
Water as needed

Soak cashews for a minimum of 4 hours to overnight. Put soaked cashews, lemon juice, sweetener, coconut oil, and vanilla in a high-speed blender such as VitaMix and process until creamy. Add water as needed; usually around ¼ cup is needed. Add the water in small amounts at a time. You don't want it to be too liquid. You can also use a food processor, but it will not be as creamy as when processed in a high-speed blender.

Note: a regular blender will not work.

Pecan Crust

1 cup flaked unsweetened coconut
1 cup pecan pieces
½ cup coconut or almond flour
2 tsp. ground cinnamon
2 Tbsp coconut nectar or pure maple syrup
5 Tbsp. coconut oil

Place all the dry ingredients in a food processor and pulse until the mixture is crumbly. Add the sweetener and coconut oil and pulse several times in short bursts until the crumbs are moist and begin to fall from the sides of the bowl. Put the crumbs into a pie plate and spread them evenly. Using your fingers, gently press the crumbs across the bottom and up the sides of the pie plate. Place in the freezer for at least 30 minutes to set. Then pour in the filling and refrigerate for at least an hour.

Shopping List	Check the Pantry
3 cups raw cashews 1 cup unsweetened coconut flakes ½ cup coconut or almond flour 1 lemon 1 cup pecan pieces	Cinnamon Coconut nectar, pure maple syrup, or liquid stevia Coconut oil Vanilla extract

Ginger Poached Pears With Hazelnuts   Serves 4

Poached pears are an elegant and healthful way to finish a meal. Reducing the flavorful poaching liquid yields a beautiful, thick sauce that sticks to the pears nicely. Top with hazelnuts and optional cocoa nibs for a bonus chocolate treat!

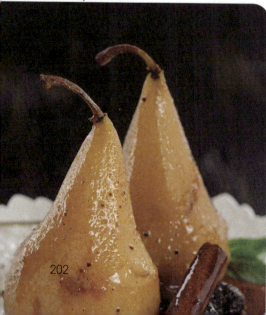

Photo by Polara Studio

Equipment

Medium to large pot
Parchment paper
Scissors
Slotted spoon

Ingredients

6 cups water
⅓ cup maple syrup (or 1 cup apple juice)
5 whole cloves
2–3 cinnamon sticks
1 tsp. vanilla extract

1 tsp. orange extract (or more vanilla extract)
Zest of 1 lemon
¼ cup ginger, coarsely chopped
4 ripe pears, peeled, cored
2 Tbsp. hazelnuts, chopped (garnish)
2 Tbsp. cocoa nibs (optional garnish)

In a large pot over medium heat, combine water, maple syrup, cloves, cinnamon sticks, vanilla extract, orange extract, lemon zest, and ginger.

As you peel and core the pears, gently slip each one into the liquid, making sure all of the pears are completely covered in poaching liquid. If you do not have a tool to core the pears, you can simply cut them in half and deseed them once they have poached and cooled.

Place a piece of parchment paper (with a hole about the size of a walnut cut in the center) over the top of the pot so that the pears stay submerged throughout cooking.

Simmer the pears on medium-low for about 30 minutes, until the pears are fork tender (but still hold their shape).

Remove the pears with a slotted spoon and lay out on a baking sheet to allow the pears to cool quickly.

Pour half of the poaching liquid in a wide skillet or sauté pan and reduce the liquid to about ½ cup, until it coats the back of a spoon.

Serve pears whole or cut in half, drenched in the reduction sauce and garnished with hazelnuts and optional cocoa nibs.

Shopping List

6-inch piece of ginger
1 lemon
4 ripe pears

Check the Pantry

Cinnamon sticks
Cocoa nibs
Hazelnuts
Maple syrup (or apple juice)
Orange extract
Vanilla extract
Whole cloves

Raspberry Linzer Bars   Yields 10 Bars

Sometimes we just need something sweet. I like to use raw honey as a main sweetener in desserts, dressings, and smoothies. When taken in small amounts, it harmonizes the liver. Honey is one of nature's finest energy-giving foods if not overused or overprocessed. Enjoy!

Coconut oil, for greasing the pan
1½ cups gluten-free all-purpose flour
¾ cup coconut sugar
½ cup plus 2 Tbsp. chopped walnuts, divided
1 Tbsp. unsweetened cocoa powder
2 tsp. freshly grated orange zest
¼ tsp. baking powder
¼ tsp. baking soda
¼ tsp. sea salt
1 tsp. ground cinnamon
¼ tsp. ground nutmeg
¼ tsp. ground cloves
1 large egg (or 1½ tsp. *Ener-G Egg Replacer* dissolved in 2 Tbsp. warm water)
2 Tbsp. olive oil
2 Tbsp. water
¾ cup seedless raspberry jam
1 Tbsp. orange juice
2 Tbsp. raw honey

Preheat the oven to 350.
    Coat a 9-by-9-inch or 7-by-11½-inch baking pan with coconut oil.
    Combine flour, sugar, walnuts (holding 2 tablespoons aside), cocoa, orange zest, baking powder, baking soda, salt, and all spices in a food processor.

Photo by Polara Studio

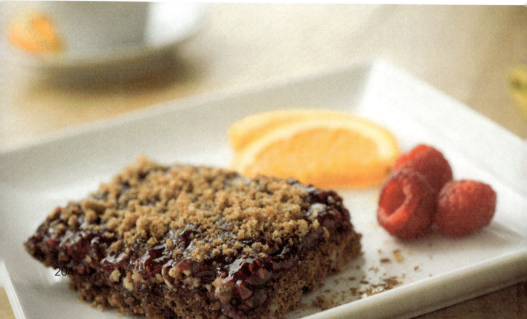

Pulse until walnuts are finely chopped. Add 1 egg (or egg replacer), olive oil, and water. Process until moistened.

Transfer the mixture to the greased pan and press into an even layer.

Bake for 20–25 minutes, until the crust becomes dry to the touch and golden.

Whisk the raspberry jam and orange juice in a bowl. Spread evenly over the crust. Sprinkle with the remaining chopped walnuts.

Bake the bars until jam bubbles, 10–15 minutes longer. Remove from oven and drizzle with honey while the bars are still very hot.

Transfer the pan to a wire rack and cool completely before cutting into bars.

Shopping List

1 large egg (or 1½ tsp. *Ener-G Egg Replacer)*
1 small orange (for zest and juice)
¾ cup seedless raspberry jam

Check the Pantry

Baking powder
Baking soda
Cinnamon
Coconut oil
Coconut sugar
Gluten-free all-purpose flour
Ground cloves
Ground nutmeg
Olive oil
Raw honey
Sea salt
Unsweetened cocoa powder
Walnuts

NOTES

Introduction
Your Diet Plan for Vibrant Health

1. Brainyquote.com, "Ralph Waldo Emerson Quotes," www
   .brainyquote.com/quotes/quotes/r/ralphwaldo105704.html
   (accessed October 8, 2014).

Chapter 1
Inflammation: Friend or Foe

1. As quoted in P. F. Louis, "Reduce Inflammation Effortlessly by
   Taking These Top Antioxidants," Naturalnews.com, July 21, 2013,
   http://www.naturalnews.com/041293_chronic_inflammation_
   immune_system_antioxidants.html (accessed October 9, 2014).

2. As quoted in Jonathan Benson, "Cholesterol Is NOT the Enemy:
   It's Inflammation That's Making You Fat and Killing You Slowly,"
   May 8, 2013, Naturalnews.com, http://www.naturalnews
   .com/040234_high_cholesterol_heart_disease_medical_myth.html
   (accessed October 15, 2014).

3. Zachary A. Marcum and Joseph T. Hanlon, "Recognizing the
   Risks of Chronic Nonsteroidal Anti-Inflammatory Drug Use in
   Older Adults," *Annals of Long Term Care* 18, no. 9 (September
   2010: 24–27.

4. David R. Hamilton, "5 Beneficial Side Effects of Kindness," Huff-
   ingtonpost.com, August 2, 2011, http://www.huffingtonpost.com/
   david-r-hamilton-phd/kindness-benefits_b_869537.html (accessed
   October 15, 2014).

5. Western Washington University, "Inflammation," http://www
   .wwu.edu/depts/healthyliving/PE511info/infection/Causes.html
   (accessed October 15, 2014).

6. U. N. Das, "Is Obesity an Inflammatory Condition?", *Nutrition* 17, no. 11–12 (November–December 2001): 953–966; P. Trayhurn and I. S. Wood, "Adipokines: Inflammation and the Pleiotropic Role of White Adipose Tissue," *British Journal of Nutrition* 92, no. 3 (September 2004): 347–355.

7. H. Florez, S. Castillo-Florez, A. Mendez, et al., "C-Reactive Protein Is Elevated in Obese Patients With the Metabolic Syndrome," *Diabetes Research and Clinical Practice* 71, no. 1 (January 2006): 92–100.

8. A. D. Pradhan, J. E. Manson, J. E. Rossouw, et al., "Inflammatory Biomarkers, Hormone Replacement Therapy, and Incident Coronary Heart Disease: Prospective Analysis From the Women's Health Initiative Observational Study," *Journal of the American Medical Association* 288, no. 8 (August 28, 2002): 980–987.

9. B. L. Stauffer, G. L. Hoetzer, D. T. Smith, and C. A. DeSouza, "Plasma C-Reactive Protein Is Not Elevated in Physically Active Postmenopausal Women Taking Hormone Replacement Therapy," *Journal of Applied Physiology* 96, no. 1 (January 2004): 143–148.

Chapter 2
Foods and Factors That Contribute to Inflammation

1. Greatest-Inspirational-Quotes.com, "Health Quotes," www .greatest-inspirational-quotes.com/health-quotes.html (accessed October 15, 2014).

2. As referenced in Jessica Levine, "The Strange Reason Diet Soda Makes You Fat," Menshealth.com, June 21, 2012, http://www. menshealth.com/weight-loss/diet-soda-fat (accessed October 15, 2014).

3. S. Liu, J. E. Manson, J. E. Buring, M. J. Stampfer, W. C. Willett, and P. M. Ridker, "Relation Between a Diet With a High Glycemic Load and Plasma Concentrations of High-Sensitivity

C-Reactive Protein in Middle-Aged Women," *American Journal of Clinical Nutrition* 75, no. 2 (March 2002): 492–498.

4. Mark Hyman, "How Diet Soda Makes You Fat (and Other Food and Diet Industry Secrets)," Huffingtonpost.com, May 7, 2013, http://www.huffingtonpost.com/dr-mark-hyman/diet-soda -health_b_2698494.html (accessed October 15, 2014).

5. Datis Kharrazian, *Why Do I Still Have Thyroid Symptoms When My Lab Tests Are Normal: A Revolutionary Breakthrough In Understanding Hashimoto's Disease and Hypothyroidism* (Carlsbad, CA: Elephant Press Books, 2010), 29.

6. Brian Foley, "Hashimoto's Thyroid Auto Immune," Health and Wellness Center, http://www.youralternativedoctor.com/hashi motos-thyroid-auto-immune/ (accessed October 15, 2014).

7. Craig A. Maxwell, "Goitrogens and Your Thyroid—the Surprising Truth You Need to Know," Askdrmaxwell.com, Sept. 9, 2013, http://www.askdrmaxwell.com/2013/09/goitrogens-and -your-thyroid-the-surprising-truth-you-need-to-know/ (accessed October 15, 2014).

8. As referenced in Mark Hyman, "Milk Is Dangerous for Your Health," Drhyman.com, November 11, 2013, http://drhyman.com/ blog/2013/10/28/milk-dangerous-health/#close (accessed October 15, 2014).

9. A. Zampelas, D. B. Panagiotakos, C. Pitsavos, C. Chrysohoou, and C. Stefanadis, "Associations Between Coffee Consumption and Inflammatory Markers in Healthy Persons: The ATTICA study," *American Journal of Clinical Nutrition* 80, No. 4 (October 2004: 862–867.

10. Mark Hyman, as quoted in Danielplan.com, "The Liquid Menace: Alcohol," http://www.danielplan.com/healthyhabits/alcohol/ (accessed October 15, 2014).

11. Mercola.com, "Engineered Poison Lurking in Your Everyday Food?", Dr. Mercola Interview With Jeffrey Smith, April 3, 2010,

http://articles.mercola.com/sites/articles/archive/2010/04/03/jeffrey-smith-interview.aspx (accessed November 12, 2014).

12. Tom Philpott, "Longest-Running GMO Safety Study Finds Tumors in Rats," MotherEarthNews.com, April/May 2013, http://www.motherearthnews.com/natural-health/gmo-safety-zmgz13amzsto.aspx#ixzz3IzXXQD3a (accessed November 14, 2014).

13. As quoted in Elisha McFarland, "The Link Between Nightshades, Chronic Pain and Inflammation," Greenmedinfo.com, April 21, 2013, http://www.greenmedinfo.com/blog/link-between-nightshades-chronic-pain-and-inflammation (accessed October 15, 2014).

14. PR Newswire, "Researchers Say Tart Cherries Have 'the Highest Anti-Inflammatory Content of Any Food,'" May 30, 2012, http://www.prnewswire.com/news-releases/researchers-say-tart-cherries-have-the-highest-anti-inflammatory-content-of-any-food-155672215.html (accessed October 15, 2014); Marco Torres, "How Tart Cherries Reduce Inflammation and Oxidative Stress," http://healthimpactnews.com/2014/how-tart-cherries-reduce-inflammation-and-oxidative-stress/ (accessed October 15, 2014).

15. SweetWater Health, "Bulletproof Food Sense iPhone App First to Detect Food Sensitivities," Sweetwaterhrv.com, July 16, 2013, http://sweetwaterhrv.com/Press/SWH%20BPE%20press%20release%20July%2016%202013.pdf (accessed October 15, 2014).

Chapter 3
Change Your Diet; Change Your Life!

1. Goodreads.com, "Hippocrates Quotes," http://www.goodreads.com/quotes/62262-let-food-be-thy-medicine-and-medicine-be-thy-food (accessed October 15, 2014).

2. Mark Hyman, *Ultra-Metabolism* (New York: Atria Books, 2006).

3. Federation of American Societies for Experimental Biology, "Antioxidant Found in Berries, Other Foods Prevents UV Skin Damage

That Leads to Wrinkles," Sciencedaily.com, April 23, 2009, http://www.sciencedaily.com/releases/2009/04/090421154318. htm (accessed October 15, 2014).

4. Lindsay Kobayashi, "To Live Longer, Eat 7 Servings of Fruits and Vegetables Per Day," (blog), Public Health Perspectives, April 8, 2014, http://blogs.plos.org/publichealth/2014/04/08/7-fruit-veg/ (accessed November 14, 2014).

5. The Nutrition Source, "Vegetables and Fruit: Get Plenty Every Day," Harvard School of Public Health, http://www.hsph.harvard. edu/nutritionsource/vegetables-full-story/ (accessed November 14, 2014).

6. Maureen Callahan, "The Fiftysomething Diet: Should You Be Juicing?", NextAvenue.org, June 30, 2014, http://www.nextavenue. org/article/2013-03/fiftysomething-diet-should-you-be-juicing (accessed November 14, 2014).

7. As referenced in Leo Galland, "Cherries for Health: Better Than Aspirin?", Huffpost.com, April 11, 2011, http://www.huffington post.com/leo-galland-md/cherry-season-fight-pain-_b_ 844654.html (accessed November 13, 2014).

8. Callahan, "The Fiftysomething Diet: Should You Be Juicing?"

9. S. V. Joseph, I. Edirisinghe, and B. M. Burton-Freeman, "Berries: Anti-Inflammatory Effects in Humans," Journal of Agricultural and Food Chemistry 62, no. 18 (March 17, 2014): 3886–3903.

10. Sally Fallon and Mary G. Enig, "The Oiling of America," Westonaprice.org, January 1, 2000, http://www.westonaprice.org/ health-topics/the-oiling-of-america/#rise (accessed October 15, 2014).

11. Stephan Guyenet, "The Diet-Heart Hypothesis: Oxidized LDL, Part 1," Whole Health Source (blog), August 3, 2009, http:// wholehealthsource.blogspot.com/2009/07/diet-heart-hypothesis-oxidized-ldl-part.html (accessed November 14, 2014).

12. Amanda Ruggeri, "Is Your Olive Oil Lying About Its Virginity?", The Cut, http://nymag.com/thecut/2014/09/your-olive-oil-lying-about-its-virginity.html (accessed November 14, 2014).

13. DrAxe.com, "Your Extra-Virgin Olive Oil Is Fake!", http://draxe.com/fake-olive-oil/ (accessed November 14, 2014).

14. MedicalNewsToday.com, "Organic Food Is More Nutritious Say EU Researchers," October 29, 2007, http://www.medicalnews-today.com/articles/86972.php (accessed November 13, 2014).

15. Kimberly Gallagher, "A Hearty Burdock Recipe, and Other Burdock Ideas," Learningherbs.com, July 1, 2010, http://learning herbs.com/remedies-recipes/burdock-recipe/ (accessed October 15, 2014).

16. Botanical Preservation Corps, "Rhodiola Root," botanical preservationcorps.com/store/rhodiola-rosea (accessed October 15, 2014).

17. Chronic Inflammation: Special Focus: Nutritional Intervention, workshop presented September, 2014, by Sally Fisher, MD.

Chapter 4
Twenty-Eight Days to Vibrant Health Recipes and Meal Plan

1. Susan Albers, "The 10 Best Healthy Eating Quotes," *Comfort Cravings* (blog), *Psychology Today*, July 13, 2011, http://psycholo-gytoday.com/blog/comfort-cravings/201107/the-10-best-healthy-eating-quotes (accessed November 7, 2014).

Sign up for the Juice Lady's free Juicy Tips
Newsletter at www.juiceladyinfo.com.

Cherie's websites

www.juiceladyinfo.com or www.juiceladycherie.com—information on juicing and weight loss

www.cheriecalbom.com

www.gococonuts.com—information about the Coconut Diet and coconut oil

The Juice Lady's health and wellness juice retreats

I invite you to join us for a week that can change your life! Our retreats offer gourmet organic raw foods with a three-day juice fast midweek. We offer interesting, informative classes in a beautiful, peaceful setting where you can experience healing and restoration of body and soul. For more information and dates for the retreats, call 866-843-8935.

The Juice Lady's health and fitness seven-week e-course

For more information, go to www.juiceladycherie.com under Weight Loss or call 866-843-8935.

Schedule a nutrition consultation with the Juice Lady team

Call 866-843-8935.

Schedule the Juice Lady to speak for your organization

Call 866-843-8935.

Books by Cherie and John Calbom

These books can be ordered at any of the websites above or by calling 866-8GETWEL (866-843-8935).

Cherie Calbom, *The Juice Lady's Big Book of Juices and Green Smoothies* (Siloam); also available in Spanish.

Cherie Calbom, *The Juice Lady's Remedies for Asthma and Allergies* (Siloam)

Cherie Calbom, *The Juice Lady's Remedies for Stress and Adrenal Fatigue* (Siloam)

Cherie Calbom, *The Juice Lady's Weekend Weight-Loss Diet* (Siloam); also available in Spanish.

Cherie Calbom, *The Juice Lady's Living Foods Revolution* (Siloam)

Cherie Calbom, *The Juice Lady's Turbo Diet* (Siloam)

Cherie Calbom, *The Juice Lady's Guide to Juicing for Health* (Avery)

Cherie Calbom and John Calbom, *Juicing, Fasting, and Detoxing for Life* (Wellness Central)

Cherie Calbom, *The Wrinkle Cleanse* (Avery)

Cherie Calbom and John Calbom, *The Coconut Diet* (Wellness Central)

Cherie Calbom, John Calbom, and Michael Mahaffey, *The Complete Cancer Cleanse* (Thomas Nelson)

Cherie Calbom, *The Ultimate Smoothie Book* (Wellness Central)

Juicers

Find out about the best juicers recommended by Cherie. Call 866-8GETWEL (866-843-8935) or visit www.juiceladyinfo.com.

Dehydrators

Find out the best dehydrators recommended by Cherie. Call 866-8GETWEL (866-843-8935) or visit www.juiceladyinfo.com.

Lymphasizer

To view the Swing Machine (lymphasizer), visit www.juiceladyinfo .com or call 866-8GETWEL (866-843-8935).

Veggie powders

To purchase or get information on Barley Max, Carrot Juice Max, and Beet Max powders, go to www.juiceladyinfo.com or call 866-8GETWEL (866-843-8935). (These powders are ideal for when you travel or when you can't get juice.)

Virgin coconut oil

For more information on virgin coconut oil, go to www.juice ladyinfo.com and www.gococonuts.com, or call 866-8GETWEL (866-843-8935). To save money, order larger sizes such as gallons or quarts, which you won't typically find in the stores.

Internal cleansing kits

The complete and comprehensive internal cleansing kit contains eighteen items for a twenty-one-day cleanse program. You get a free colon cleanse kit, along with Liver-Gallbladder Rejuvenator, Friendly Bacteria Replenisher, Parasite Cleanser, Lung Rejuvenator, Kidney and Bladder Rejuvenator, Blood and Skin Rejuvenator, and Lymph Rejuvenator. See www.juiceladycherie.com for more information. You may order the cleansing products and get the 10 percent discount by calling 866-843-8935.

Berry Breeze

Keep your produce fresher longer and your fridge smelling fresh too. It can save you up to $2,200 a year from lost produce. Go to www .juiceladycherie.com.

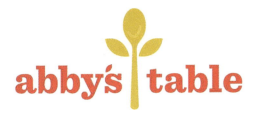

Sign up for Chef Abby's weekly inspiration newsletter for recipes, life-styles tips, and more cooking resources: www.abbys-table.com

Chef Abby's website with more recipes, weekly blog tips, and events: www.abbys-table.com

Contact Chef Abby at info@abbys-table.com.

For food lifestyle classes and consultations, contact Abby at (503) 828-7662.

For private group classes and hands-on dinner parties, contact Abby at info@abbys-table.com or (503) 828-7662.

Facebook: search for Abby's Table, Portland, OR

Instagram: abbycookswith

Pinterest: Abby's Table

Twitter: #abbystable

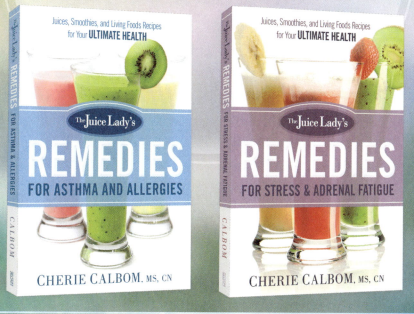

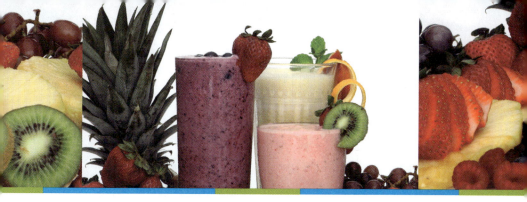

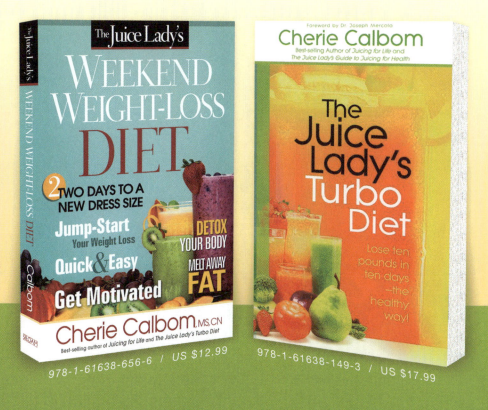

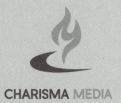